JN299521

プライマリー薬学シリーズ 1
薬学英語入門
CD 付

日本薬学会編

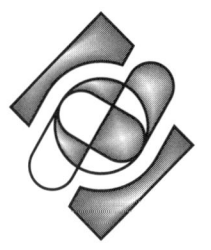

東京化学同人

まえがき

　本書は日本薬学会の薬学教育カリキュラムを検討する協議会が定めた"薬学準備教育ガイドライン（例示）"（2002年8月）に準拠してつくられた薬学生のための英語教科書です．ガイドラインには"(1) 人と文化", "(2) 薬学英語入門", "(3)～(6) 薬学の基礎としての物理，化学，生物，数学・統計"などについて，それぞれの一般目標と到達目標が示されています．外国語は，そのうち"(1) 人と文化"の到達目標達成のための学問領域として例示されています．しかし，英語については，独立した項目"(2) 薬学英語入門"として一般目標と到達目標が明記されています（前見返し参照）．さらに，先に示した(3)～(6)などと同等に扱われているのを見るならば，英語が薬学の基礎として重要であることがわかるでしょう．

　高校までに勉強してきた英語と"薬学英語入門"で求められる英語はどのように違うのでしょうか．それは"一般目標"を見るとよくわかります．大きく異なっているのは，対象が"薬学を中心とした自然科学の分野で必要とされる英語"であることです．具体的には"読む"，"書く"，"聞く・話す"それぞれに"到達目標"が設定されています．これらの目標を達成するための教材として，この教科書にはさまざまな工夫が盛り込まれています．まず，各章の初めにはその章の目標（Objectives）として到達目標（SBOs）が割当てられていますから，必ず確認して予習に臨んでください．Readingの英文は，"薬学教育モデル・コアカリキュラム"から満遍なくトピックを選び出し，専門科目の教科書や官公庁のホームページから原文のまま転載したものです．難解と思われる単語などには説明を加えました．練習問題も豊富に設けてあります．Reading Comprehension（内容確認），Grammatical Rule（文法事項の確認），Writing（作文），Medical Vocabulary（医学用語），Listening/Speaking（聞く・話す）それぞれの練習問題に自分はなぜ取組んでいるのかを常に意識してください．章の最後にはCOLUMN（コラム）が設けてあり，薬学に関するホットなニュースをお伝えします．巻末には，Appendixとして発音ルール表，発音記号一覧表，ライティングのヒントが付いています．高校までの英語の復習として上手に使ってください．

　この教科書は，日本薬学英語研究会（JAPE）と日本薬学会薬学教育部会との協働でつくられたものです．JAPEは薬学部の英語教員と薬学英語に関心の深い専門教員により2007年3月に設立され，大学の垣根を越えた薬学生のための英語教育情報交換ネットワークとして意見交換，大学訪問，研究発表などの活動を行っています．すでに2冊の薬学英語テキストも出版しています（"薬学英語1, 2", 成美堂, 2009）．

　今回，"プライマリー薬学シリーズ1"としてこのテキストを作成するに当たっては，多くの方々のお世話になりました．特にJAPEと薬学教育部会のコラボレーションの実現に向けご支援くださった東京化学同人編集部の住田六連氏と丸山　潤氏に深く感謝申し上げます．

2011年1月

"薬学英語入門"編集委員一同

第1巻　薬学英語入門

編集委員

入江　徹美	熊本大学大学院生命科学研究部 教授，薬学博士
金子　利雄	日本大学薬学部 教授，文学修士，M.A.(英語学)
河野　　円	明治大学総合数理学部 教授，M.A.(第二言語習得)
Eric M. Skier	東京薬科大学薬学部 准教授，M.A.(英語教授法)
竹内　典子	明治薬科大学薬学部 教授，文学修士
中村　明弘	昭和大学薬学部 教授，薬学博士
堀内　正子*	昭和薬科大学薬学部 准教授，修士(英語教育)

*責任者

執筆者

板垣　　正	日本大学薬学部 講師，Ph.D.
市川　　厚	武庫川女子大学薬学部 教授，京都大学名誉教授，薬学博士
入江　徹美	熊本大学大学院生命科学研究部 教授，薬学博士
入倉　　充	第一薬科大学 教授，博士(薬学)
小澤孝一郎	広島大学大学院医歯薬保健学研究院 教授，薬学博士
金子　利雄	日本大学薬学部 教授，文学修士，M.A.(英語学)
上村　直樹	東京理科大学薬学部 教授，博士(薬学)
河野　　円	星薬科大学薬学部 教授，M.A.(第二言語習得)
木内　祐二	昭和大学薬学部 教授，医学博士
木津　純子	慶應義塾大学薬学部 教授，博士(薬学)
小林　　文	昭和大学薬学部 助教，修士(薬学)
齋藤　弘明	日本大学薬学部 助教，修士(薬学)
笹津　備規	東京薬科大学 学長，薬学博士
Eric M. Skier	東京薬科大学薬学部 准教授，M.A.(英語教授法)
須川久美子	昭和薬科大学 非常勤講師，修士(文学)
竹内　典子	明治薬科大学薬学部 教授，文学修士
田沢　恭子	明治薬科大学 非常勤講師，修士(人文科学)
寺田　　弘	東京理科大学薬学部 教授，徳島大学名誉教授，薬学博士
富岡　　清	同志社女子大学薬学部 特任教授，京都大学名誉教授，薬学博士
中村　明弘	昭和大学薬学部 教授，薬学博士
西村　月満	北里大学一般教育部 教授，文学修士，M.A.(英語学)
平田　收正	大阪大学大学院薬学研究科 教授，薬学博士
堀内　正子	昭和薬科大学薬学部 准教授，修士(英語教育)
山田　　惠	北海道薬科大学薬学部 教授，博士(文学)

執 筆 分 担

1. Reading, 2. Reading Comprehension：

1章　金　子	2章　堀　内	3章　金　子	4章　山　田
5章　須　川	6章　河　野	7章　齋　藤	8章　竹　内
9章　山　田	10章　竹　内	11章　板　垣	12章　河　野
13章　竹　内	14章　堀　内	15章　田　沢	16章　西　村
17章　堀　内	18章　須　川	19章　田　沢	20章　金子，小林

3. Grammatical Rule： 1〜20章　金　子
4. Writing： 1〜20章　河　野
5. Medical Vocabulary： 1〜20章　竹　内
6. Listening/Speaking： 1〜20章　Skier

COLUMN 執筆分担

1章　木　内	2章　小　澤	5章　市　川	6章　寺　田
7章　富　岡	8章　平　田	9章　笹　津	10章　木　内
11章　寺　田	12章　富　岡	13章　笹　津	14章　平　田
16章　入　江	17章　木　津	18章　中　村	19章　入　倉
20章　上　村			

テキストの使用にあたって

　まずはじめに，テキストの見返しにある薬学準備教育ガイドライン（例示）の日本語と英語を読み比べてみてください．英語訳はこのテキストをつくるにあたって JAPE（日本薬学英語研究会）が翻訳したものです．英語訳の方がより明確になっていることがわかるでしょう．たとえば，一般目標（GIO）の英語訳では，"Students should acquire ～"，【読む】到達目標（SBO）2 では，"Can explain ～ in Japanese or English." と，下線の部分が書き加えられています．また，"読む"，"書く"，"聞く"，"話す" という 4 技能をバランスよく高めるために，さまざまな工夫がされています．もちろん原則は，高校までの英語の基礎を修得しているという前提ですが，復習の機会も提供します．これらを十分に理解して，目標達成のための道具としてこのテキストを最大限に有効活用して下さい．

【本書の構成】

　見返しに示したように，薬学英語に関する SBO は包括的ですので，これを達成するためには，さまざまな場面で繰返し学習・練習することが必要です．そこで本書は，SBO ごとではなく，自然科学的な英文例（Reading）を学びながら，各 SBO を修得できるように構成してあります．

　各章の最初に掲げた **Objectives** は，その章を学ぶことにより達成できる具体的な目標です．その行末にはその目標を包含する SBO を示しました．たとえば，1 章の目標（Objectives）の 1 番目は，SBO 2 に関するもので，SBO 2 "Can explain the content of simple written passages in English or Japanese" は "Explain what the White Coat Ceremony is in English or Japanese" と Reading のトピックスに直接かかわる内容に書き換えられています．

　欄外の **対応 SBO** は，その章のどの部分がその SBO の達成に役立つかを示しました．たとえば，SBO 2 の能力は 1 章の "Reading" と "Reading Comprehension"，そして "Grammatical Rule" を学ぶことにより高められます．

　各節の組立ては以下のようになっています．

1. Reading　　各章のトピックは "薬学教育モデル・コアカリキュラム"（主として 4 年生までに修得する内容）の A, B, C1 ～ C18 を順番に 20 に分割し，おのおのの領域からより具体的なテーマを一つ選び出したもので，それに則した英文を掲載しました．皆さんが初めて目にする英文も多いかもしれません．難解と思われる単語には，各ページの左右に注をつけてありますから，楽しみながら読み進んでください．

2. Reading Comprehension　　内容確認の問題です．"英語の質問に英語で答える"，"英語の質問に日本語で答える"，"英語要約文の英単語穴埋め"，"英文内容の真偽"，"英単語の英語定義の選択" などさまざまな練習問題を解いて，正確に内容が把握できているかどうかを確認します．

3. Grammatical Rule　　文法事項の確認問題です．高校までに習った文法事項の確認をすると同時に，自然科学の英文で用いられる特徴を各章 1 項目に絞って解説します．

4. Writing　英作文の問題です．ここでは，日本語を英語にするだけではなく，自分の考えを述べることにも注目しています．

5. Medical Vocabulary　医学用語や医療用語を覚えるための問題です．そのほとんどはこれまでふれることのなかった用語でしょう．少しずつ，系統的に覚えていきましょう．

6. Listening/Speaking　最近は，薬学部にも短期・長期で外国の研究者や研究生がやって来ることが増えているようです．また，日本から外国の薬学部に見学実習に行く人たちも増えています．

　1章から20章まで，アメリカの姉妹校から二人の薬学生が短期留学で日本にやって来たという想定でストーリーが展開します．最初は単語レベルの聞きとりから文の聞きとり，最後は学内放送や二人の会話の聞きとりまでさまざまな問題を用意しています．楽しみながら取組んでください．そして，実際に使ってみてください．

　左のアイコンはその節の音声が付属のCDに収録されていることを示します．1章～10章のReadingと1章～20章のListening/SpeakingがCDに収録されています．何度も繰返し，聞く練習をしましょう．また，少し遅れて自分でも声を出して追いかけていきましょう．

目　　次

第 1 巻 薬 学 英 語 入 門

Chapter 1　White Coat Ceremonies（白衣授与式）……………………………2
Chapter 2　International Pharmaceutical Students' Federation（世界薬学生連盟）……8
Chapter 3　The Story Behind the Discovery of the Fullerene
　　　　　　　　　　　　　　　　　　（フラーレン発見の裏話）……14
Chapter 4　Acid Rain（酸性雨）………………………………………………20
Chapter 5　DNA（デオキシリボ核酸）………………………………………26
Chapter 6　The Nobel Prize in Chemistry (2001)（2001 年ノーベル化学賞）…………32
Chapter 7　The Race to Synthesize Taxol（タキソール合成競争）……………38
Chapter 8　Copper（銅）………………………………………………………44
Chapter 9　Bacteria, Viruses, and Antibiotics（細菌，ウイルスと抗生物質）…………50
Chapter 10　Living with Parkinson's Disease（パーキンソン病と共に生きる）…………56
Chapter 11　The Science of Drug Abuse & Addiction
　　　　　　　　　　　　　（薬物乱用と薬物中毒にいたる仕組み）……62
Chapter 12　Allergies（アレルギー）……………………………………………68
Chapter 13　*E. coli*（大腸菌）……………………………………………………74
Chapter 14　Report Calls for Clean Up of World's Dirtiest Dozen
　　　　　　　　　　　（報告書：世界最悪 12 地域の汚染浄化を要請）……81
Chapter 15　A Drug's Life（薬の一生）…………………………………………88
Chapter 16　Anti-Cancer Drugs（抗癌剤）………………………………………94
Chapter 17　Medicines for the Future（未来の薬）……………………………100
Chapter 18　Nanotechnology and Drug Delivery（ナノテクノロジーと薬物送達）……106
Chapter 19　Inside Clinical Trials: Testing Medical Products in People
　　　　　　　　　　　　　（治験の内情：医薬品をヒトで検証）……112
Chapter 20　Self-Medication（セルフメディケーション）………………………118

Appendix
1. 発音ルール表 …………………………………………………………………126
2. 発音記号（phonetic symbol）一覧表 ………………………………………127
3. ライティングのヒント ………………………………………………………128

Introduction to Pharmacy English

Chapter 1

White Coat Ceremonies

Objectives

After studying this chapter, you should be able to:
- Explain what the White Coat Ceremony is in English or Japanese. [SBO 2]
- Describe the high ideals as a student of pharmacy in the U.S. in English or Japanese. [SBO 2]
- Utilize one of the basic grammatical rules, apposition, for reading and writing. [SBOs 2, 4, 5]
- Rewrite short Japanese sentences about Japanese culture and campus life into English without grammatical errors. [SBO 5]
- Write a self-introduction in English. [SBO 6]
- Define basic terms pertaining to pharmacy. [SBO 3]
- Tell the difference between sounds in spoken English. [SBO 10]

対応 SBO
SBO 2

1・1 Reading

> 日本の6年制薬学教育は，医療を担う薬剤師としての"知識・技能・態度"を養うことを目的とする．では，医療人としての態度を養うためにはどうしたらよいだろうか．米国の Pharm. D. Program は，基礎教育（最短2年）を終えた者のための薬学専門課程（4年制）である．米国薬剤師会が紹介している一般向け広報ホームページをのぞいてみよう．入学時に行われる厳かなセレモニーから薬剤師になるという強い自覚，責任感，誇りが共感できよう．

Track 1

Description of Activity

In an effort to demonstrate professionalism, many colleges of pharmacy have implemented a White Coat Ceremony for new students. These ceremonies are often held early in the students' experience, for example during orientation, the first day of class, or some time during their first semester. Some schools hold the ceremony in the third year as students move from the didactic to the clinical portion of their Pharm. D. Degree program. Each ceremony should be developed around the unique needs

implement 実行する
White Coat Ceremony
白衣授与式

didactic (portion)
講義期間

of each school. The White Coat ceremony may be planned during the day or in the evening. Often the ceremony is held in conjunction with a social event, such as a lunch, dinner, or reception. It is a time of celebration and remembrance. A keynote speaker may be invited as well as other prominent members of the community, such as legislators, campus administrators, or the president of the state pharmacy association. Many schools also include parents, spouses, current students, and faculty members in the celebration. In addition to giving each student a new white coat, the ceremony may include a time for students to recite *the Oath of the Pharmacist* or *the Pledge of Professionalism*. Several schools have the new student class write its own oath or pledge to be recited at the ceremony.

Rationale

The "white coat" is a powerful symbol of the awesome responsibility that pharmacists have as healthcare providers. The presentation of the white coat to new students represents their passage into the pharmacy profession with all the opportunities and responsibilities associated with professionalism. The ceremony also provides an opportunity for the class to come together (to celebrate a significant event together) for the first time which is quite memorable for many students. Having family members and other important individuals participate also adds to this event.

The Pledge of Professionalism

As a student of pharmacy, I believe there is a need to build and reinforce a professional identity founded on integrity, ethical behavior and honor. This development, a vital process in my education, will help to ensure that I am true to the professional relationship I establish between myself and society as I become a member of the pharmacy community.

Integrity will be an essential part of my everyday life and I will pursue all academic and professional endeavors with honesty and commitment to service.

To accomplish this goal of professional development, as a student of pharmacy I will:

A. **DEVELOP** a sense of loyalty and duty to the profession by contributing to the well-being of others and by enthusiastically accepting the responsibility and accountability for membership in the profession.

B. **FOSTER** professional competency through life-long learning. I will strive for high ideals, teamwork, and unity within the profession in order to provide optimal patient care.

C. **SUPPORT** my colleagues by actively encouraging personal commitment to the Oath of a Pharmacist and the Code of Ethics for Pharmacists as set forth by the profession.

D. **DEDICATE** my life and practice to excellence. This will require an ongoing reassessment of personal and professional values.

E. **MAINTAIN** the highest ideals and professional attributes to insure and facilitate the covenantal relationship required of the pharmaceutical care giver.

　The profession of pharmacy is one that demands adherence to a set of ethical principles. These high ideals are necessary to insure the quality of care extended to the patients I serve. As a student of pharmacy, I believe this does not start with graduation; rather it begins with my membership in this professional college community. Therefore, I will strive to uphold this pledge as I advance toward full membership in the profession.

出　典：©2010 American Pharmacists Association, http://www.pharmacist.com/AM/Template.cfm?Section＝White_Coat_Ceremonies1（2010年12月1日現在）より許可を得て転載．

1・2　Reading Comprehension

▶ **Question**　Answer the following questions in English.

1. What is the White Coat Ceremony?

   _____

2. When are the White Coat Ceremonies held?

   _____

3. What does the White Coat imply?

   _____

4. You will wear a white coat in the laboratory and pharmacists in the hospital or drugstore must wear the same white coat. However, the latter means a lot. What is the main difference between the two white coats?

   _____

5. The phrase "a set of ethical principles" seems to imply the four principles of medical ethics. Consult a medical dictionary or website, and answer in Japanese.

   (a) （　　　　　　　　）の原則　　(b) （　　　　　　　　）の原則

   (c) （　　　　　　　　）の原則　　(d) （　　　　　　　　）の原則

1・3　Grammatical Rule: 同格 (Apposition)

同格とは "ある語句のより詳細な情報を後ろに並べる表現法" である．自然科学の英文では，新出用語，難解な専門用語の後に，その用語を説明する同格表現が使われていることが多く，大変助かることがある．難しい語に出会ってもけっして慌てることなく，後続文を読むことである．きっと解釈の手がかりが見つかるはずである．

同格表現には，以下の4種類がおもに使われる．

(1) カンマを用いた同格

　　There are two genes, *BRCA1 and BRCA2*.

(2) or を用いた同格

　　Species, *or groups of the same creature*, change over time.

(3) 前置詞 of を用いた同格

　　I have a good idea *of preventing a new flu*.

(4) 接続詞 that を用いた同格

　　Everyone knows the fact *that DNA has a double helix structure*.

では，本文中の次の例文を見てみよう．同格表現がどこに使われているか考えてみよう．

> This development, a vital process in my education, will help to ensure that I am true to the professional relationship...

1・4 Writing

対応 SBO: SBOs 5,6

1. Grammatical Rule を参考にして以下の作文をしなさい．

   a) 納豆（natto）は発酵した大豆（fermented soybeans）で，朝食にしばしば出される日本の伝統食です．

   _____

   _____

   b) 週末はインドからの交換留学生（an exchange student）の Mohamed を浅草見物に連れていく予定です．

   _____

   _____

   c) 大学の学生食堂（student cafeteria）の"仲間"でお茶しましょう．緑の屋根があるのですぐわかります．

   _____

   _____

2. 隣の席の人を英文 3 文以上で紹介しなさい．文ごとに改行しないこと．

   _____

   _____

   _____

   _____

1・5 Medical Vocabulary

対応 SBO: SBO 3

Match the following terms with their definitions and write the appropriate letter (a〜e) to the right of each term.

1. clinical　　　　_____
2. pharmacy　　　_____
3. pharmaceutical　_____
4. pharmacist　　　_____
5. healthcare　　　_____

a. one who prepares, sells, or dispenses drugs
b. relating to medicinal drugs
c. the organized provision of medical care to individuals or a community
d. relating to the observation and treatment of actual patients
e. the science or practice of the preparation and dispensing of medical drugs

1・6 Listening/Speaking

▶ **Dictation**   Listen to the following conversation and fill in the blanks.

対応 SBO
SBO 10

At a Welcome Party in the Student Hall.

Prof. Nagai: Good morning everyone. Today, I am happy to introduce <u>you to</u> two visiting students: Lisa <u>Yamanaka and Bruce</u> Chen. They are from our (　　　　　　) in America.

Lisa Yamanaka: Hi.

Bruce Chen: Hi, everyone.

Prof. Nagai: First, Lisa and Bruce, please introduce yourselves. Everyone listen (　　　　　).

Lisa Yamanaka: I'm Lisa Yamanaka and this is my first time to Japan. I look (　　　　　　) being here. Thanks.

Bruce Chen: Hi, my name's Bruce and this is also my first time to Japan. I am really excited! I <u>want to</u> go to Akihabara!

Prof. Nagai: And we are (　　　　) to have you. They will be studying here for the next six weeks, so please don't be a (　　　　) to them. OK?

Now work with your partner and try to say the above dialog (in natural English).

Naturally Spoken English Notes:
　you to = youda　　Yamanaka and Bruce = Yamanaka'nBruce
　want to = wanna

COLUMN

医療人に必要な知識・技能・態度
(Knowledge, Skills, Attitudes and Behavior Required Medical Staff)

　医療を担う医師，薬剤師，看護師などの医療専門職にとって，病気・患者，治療・ケアなどに関するばく大な専門的知識，医療のプロとしての診断や治療・ケアにかかわるさまざまな専門技能，患者や医療スタッフとのコミュニケーションや倫理観，責任感といった態度，すなわち医療人としての"知識"，"技能"，"態度"の三領域がいずれも重要である．医療人に求められる使命は，なによりも専門的な知識とプロの技能を用いて治るべき患者を確実に治すことである．これを"Scienceとしての医療"ということができる．それとともに治療が不可能あるいは治療が困難な患者が，私たち医療人に出会うことにより，少しでも希望をもつことができる，さらには人生の最後に穏やかな気持ちになってもらうことも大切な使命である．こうした医療は"Artとしての医療"（日野原重明）ということが

できるであろう．患者ごとに自分の病気や人生にそれぞれの思いをもっている．医療職を目指す諸君には，患者の思いを実現する患者中心の医療の担い手として，医療人として求められる知識・技能・態度をバランスよく学習し，身につけてもらいたい．

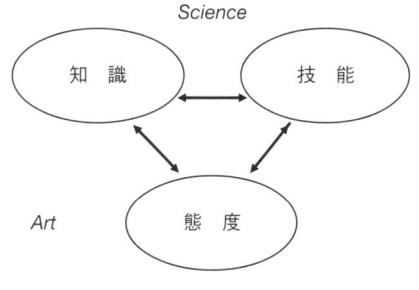

（木内祐二）

Chapter 2
International Pharmaceutical Students' Federation

Objectives

After studying this chapter, you should be able to:
- Explain what IPSF is in English or Japanese. [SBO 2]
- Describe the purpose and activities of IPSF in English or Japanese. [SBO 2]
- Utilize one of the basic grammatical rules, phrases, for reading and writing. [SBOs 2, 4, 5]
- List basic measurements and numbers related to the natural sciences. [SBO 7]
- Explain basic terms pertaining to parts of the body. [SBO 3]
- Tell the difference between sounds in spoken English. [SBO 10]
- Ask and answer questions that come up in an English conversation between two pharmacy students. [SBO 12]
- Correctly pronounce parts of the body. [SBO 13]

対応 SBO
SBO 2

2・1 Reading

> "あなたは何人？"と問われたらどう答えるだろうか．私たちは地球市民だ．地球に住むものは，人も動物も皆，一つの船に乗り合わせた運命共同体なのだ．自分の周りや日本のことを考えることは大切だが，世界レベルで物事を考えることも必要だ．世界の薬学生は何を考え，何を学び，どんな活動をしているのだろうか．ここでは，世界薬学生連盟のホームページをのぞいてみよう．そう，これはあなたに向けて語られている．

Track 3

IPSF 世界薬学生連盟

graduate 卒業生

advocacy 弁護，支持

public health 公衆衛生

initiative 構想，戦略

The International Pharmaceutical Students' Federation (IPSF) was founded in 1949 by eight pharmacy student associations in London. The Federation now represents approximately 350,000 pharmacy students and recent graduates in 70 countries worldwide. IPSF is the leading international advocacy organisation for pharmacy students promoting improved public health through provision of information, education, networking, and a range of publications and professional activities.

IPSF initiatives focus mainly on the areas of public health and pharmacy education and professional development. Initiatives include public health campaigns, research on issues in pharmacy education and workforce development, the Student Exchange Programme, organising international and regional congresses and symposia, and publication of the IPSF News Bulletin, Newsletter and educational supplement *Phuture*.

IPSF holds Official Relations with the World Health Organization (WHO), Operational Relations with the United Nations Educational, Scientific, and Cultural Organization (UNESCO), and Roster Consultative Status with the Economic Social Council of the United Nations (UN ECOSOC). IPSF works in close collaboration with the International Pharmaceutical Federation (FIP). The IPSF Secretariat is supported and hosted by the FIP in The Hague, the Netherlands.

Pharmacy Education

Education plays an extremely important role in preparing pharmacy students for practice and other professional activities. It serves to ensure adequate and appropriate competence, knowledge, skills, attitudes and behaviour required of pharmacists in order to contribute to communities and health systems in the best possible ways. It is the foundation of nurturing the 7＋1 star pharmacist as recognised by the World Health Organization (WHO) and the International Pharmaceutical Federation (FIP).

The seven roles of the pharmacist are: caregiver, decision-maker, communicator, manager, life-long learner, teacher and leader, with the added function of the pharmacist as a researcher.

IPSF is committed to ensuring quality pharmacy education. It is IPSF's stand that students are an important stakeholder of the profession, and thus should be involved in and contribute towards the development and presentation of their education and profession. The Federation strives to provide pharmacy students around the globe with avenues to broaden their knowledge base and encourages member associations to be proactive in improving pharmacy education.

TOBACCO ALERT CAMPAIGN

Following the proactive action of the World Health Organization (WHO) to adopt smoking as one of its main targets for action, IPSF elected to implement a campaign aiming to help stop this epidemic in all facets of the population. The IPSF Tobacco Alert Campaign was officially launched during the 1998 IPSF Congress in Helsinki, Finland, and has since grown to be one of the most popular initiatives of the Federation.

It is widely known that tobacco is a major factor in numerous health conditions for both smokers and non-smokers. As we find out more and understand the consequences of tobacco use on the passive smoker, the need to create tobacco-free public areas becomes extremely important. It is in this context that IPSF proposes a campaign to transform your university into a healthier environment. We cannot forget that as future health professionals, we have responsibilities in this area and we should be, whenever possible, an example to the public. With this in mind, IPSF is encouraging all Faculties of Pharmacy worldwide to step up and make all pharmacy premises, related events, activities, parties, celebrations, and gatherings tobacco free.

出典：©2007 International Pharmaceutical Students' Federation, http://www.ipsf.org/about_ipsf.php, http://www.ipsf.org/pharmacy_education.php, http://www.ipsf.org/public_health.php（2010年12月1日現在）．

2・2 Reading Comprehension

▶ **Question** Answer the following questions in English.

対応 SBO
SBOs 2,4,5

1. When and by whom was IPSF started?
   _____

2. How many pharmacy students does IPSF represent? And are they from a few countries?
   _____

3. What is IPSF's aim?
   _____

4. What is the 7+1 star pharmacist? Write the 7+1 roles of the pharmacist in Japanese.

   (1) _____   (2) _____
   (3) _____   (4) _____
   (5) _____   (6) _____
   (7) _____   (8) _____

5. Why has IPSF selected the "Tobacco Alert Campaign" as one of their activities?
   _____

2・3 Grammatical Rule: 句 (Phrases)

対応 SBO
SBOs 2,4,5

　文は，接辞，語幹，語，句，節という構成要素から成り立っている．ちょうど，物質が原子や分子から成り立っているのと同様である．文を正しく理解するためには，文を構成している構成要素とそれらの間の関係を理解することが必要である．この章では句について考えてみよう．

　句とは，"2語以上の語が集まって一つの意味単位を構成し，かつ，それ自身が主語＋動詞の形式を備えていないもの"のことである．その集まりの中心となる語の種類によって，名詞句，動詞句，形容詞句，副詞句，前置詞句，不定詞句，分詞句などとよんでいるが，大切なことは，どこまでが句であるかを正しく理解できることである．会話の息をつくところでもあるので，間違えると意味が正しく伝わらなくなるので気をつけよう．

　では，文中の次の例文を用いて，句の切れ目に斜線を入れてみよう．

　Following the proactive action of the WHO to adopt smoking as one of its main targets for action, IPSF elected to implement a campaign aiming to help stop this epidemic in all facets of the population.

2. International Pharmaceutical Students' Federation

対応 SBO
SBO 7

2・4 Writing

温度に関する表現，および分数の読み方を学ぼう．

摂氏 Celsius〔℃〕と華氏 Fahrenheit〔℉〕の関係は次式で表される．

$$[°F] = [°C] \times \frac{9}{5} + 32$$

▶ **Question** 次の問題に英語で答えなさい．

1. What water temperature do you prefer when you take a bath?

   _____

2. What is the boiling point of water in degrees Fahrenheit?

   _____

3. When a person has influenza, what will his/her temperature be in degrees Fahrenheit?

   _____

対応 SBO
SBOs 3,13

2・5 Medical Vocabulary

Write the name of each numbered part on the corresponding line.

(1) _____   (2) _____

(3) _____   (4) _____

(5) _____   (6) _____

(7) _____   (8) _____

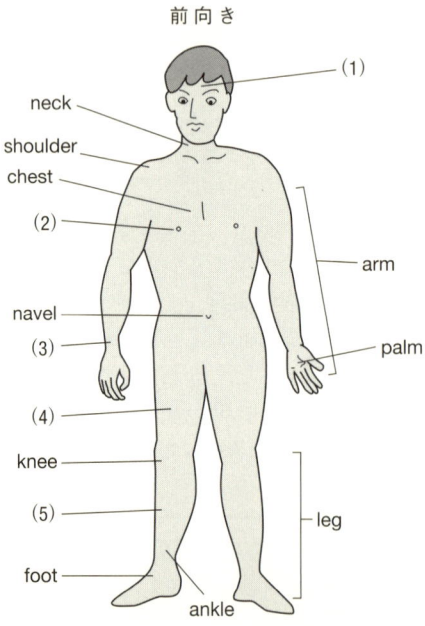
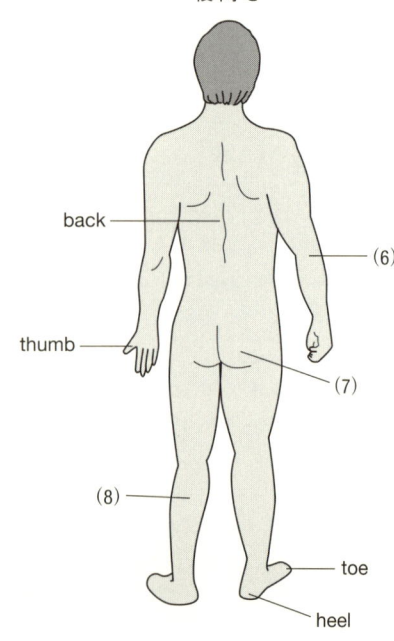

2·6 Listening/Speaking

▶ **Dictation** Listen to the following conversation and fill in the blanks.

対応 SBO
SBOs 10,12

CD Track 4

At the Cafeteria

Yoko Kimura: Hi, I'm Yoko. (   ) are...?
Lisa Yamanaka: My name is Lisa. Nice to meet you.
Yoko Kimura: (   ). Can I ask you a question?
Lisa Yamanaka: Sure.
Yoko Kimura: Are you a (   )?
Lisa Yamanaka: Not yet. I am a 4th-year Pharm.D. student visiting from California.
Yoko Kimura: Oh, I'm still a (   ).
Lisa Yamanaka: So, how many more years will you study pharmacy?
Yoko Kimura: In Japan, we have to study for six years. So, I have (   ).
Lisa Yamanaka: That's not bad. This is my (   ) year of study.
Yoko Kimura: Eight years! That's a long time! You (   )!

Now work with your partner and try to say the above dialog (in natural English), but use your own words. For example, instead of "Yoko," use your own name.

Naturally Spoken English Notes:

and you = andju   nice to meet you = nicetameetcha   can I = kennai

COLUMN

ますます広がる，地域における薬剤師の役割

　薬剤師は，保険調剤，セルフメディケーション，在宅医療などを通して，また，薬事衛生の専門家として，禁煙活動の支援（禁煙指導員），ドーピング禁止活動の支援，災害時医療への支援参加など，幅広く地域医療に貢献する活動を行っている．これら地域における薬剤師の活動の一つとして，**学校薬剤師**があげられる．学校薬剤師とは，学校保健安全法に"大学以外の学校には，学校医，学校歯科医及び学校薬剤師を置くものとする."と規定されているものであり，学校設置者から委任委嘱される役職である．その職務は学校の環境衛生に関する検査と維持改善についての助言指導をはじめさまざまなものがあるが，最近では児童・生徒への"喫煙，飲酒，薬物乱用の防止"教育も行われている．さらに2008, 2009年度の中学校と高等学校の学習指導要領改訂により，保健体育（保健分野）に"喫煙，飲酒，薬物乱用の防止"に関する内容に加え，"医薬品の適正使用"が必須の内容として盛り込まれ，薬剤師は学校における児童・生徒への教育という新しい役割を通し，さらに幅広く地域に貢献して行くこととなる．

（小澤孝一郎）

Chapter 3
The Story Behind the Discovery of the Fullerene

Objectives

After studying this chapter, you should be able to:

- Read simple written sentences and identify the main idea in a timely fashion. [SBO 1]
- Explain how fullerenes were discovered in English or Japanese. [SBO 3]
- Correctly explain English written for the sciences in Japanese or English. [SBO 4]
- Utilize one of the basic grammatical rules, coordinate conjunctions, for reading and writing. [SBOs 2, 4, 5]
- Rewrite short Japanese sentences about Japanese culture and campus life into English without grammatical errors. [SBO 5]
- Explain the content of English, including technical terms, related to pharmacy in Japanese or English. [SBO 3]
- Tell the difference between sounds in spoken English. [SBO 10]
- Correctly pronounce parts of the body. [SBO 13]

対応 SBO
SBOs 1,3,4

3・1 Reading

> 1996年，フラーレンの発見により Smalley ら外国人研究者にノーベル化学賞が授与された．しかし，それよりも前にその存在を予言した日本人化学者がいた．邦文で発表した論文が明暗を分けたのである．また，データの意味を正しく理解せず，大発見を逸してしまった事例もある．これらのエピソードを読んで，研究とはどうあるべきかを考えてみよう．

Track 5

molecule 分子

Osawa's Prediction of Fullerenes

In the past, carbon molecules were believed to have three basic shapes: diamond-type, graphite-type and amorphous-type. In September 1984, however, Richard E. Smalley and Robert F. Curl of Rice University, and Harold W. Kroto of the University of Sussex in England discovered the existence of the fourth type of carbon molecule. These soccer-ball-shaped molecules, created by linking together 60 carbon atoms,

atom 原子

represented a closed-shell structure comprising twelve equilateral pentagons and twenty equilateral hexagons. Smalley and two other researchers named such structures fullerenes (a generic term for carbon-family compounds consisting of such a closed-shell structure, including C_{60}). The three scholars were awarded the Nobel Prize in chemistry in 1996.

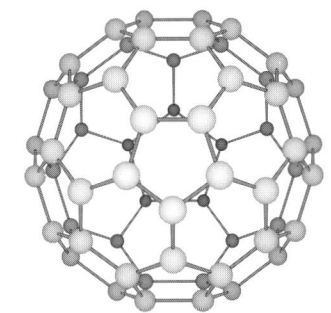

Fullerene

It should be noted that a Japanese scholar had predicted the existence of fullerenes. In 1971, Toyohashi University of Technology Professor Eiji Osawa (then an assistant researcher at Kyoto University) predicted the existence of a soccer-ball-shaped C_{60} molecule in his book *Properties of Aromatics* (Kagakudojin), coauthored with Kinki University Professor Zenichi Yoshida. Osawa later told Smalley that his book had generated almost no reaction partly because it was written in Japanese.

In response, Smalley noted that the new type of carbon molecules attracted considerable attention because they were named fullerenes after R. Buckminster Fuller, who was well known for his design of the geodesic dome structure called "buckyballs." He and his group also insisted on calling the carbon nanotube to be described later as a "Bucky tube." We often see international competition in the world of scientists with respect to naming a new discovery (i.e., becoming the godfather of discovered materials or phenomena), as this conveys a special cachet in terms of the originality of the discovery.

Discovery of Fullerenes

At the time, Smalley and Curl had been searching for clusters with a specific molecular weight through a process of bombarding silicon and germanium with laser beams and analyzing the evaporating clusters

3. The Story Behind the Discovery of the Fullerene

mass spectroscopy 質量分析
interstellar matter 星間物質
joint research 共同研究

(groups of atoms) by mass spectroscopy. Kroto was working on interstellar matter (matter existing in the near-vacuum of outer space) that attracted his attention, and asked Smalley to initiate a joint research program to artificially create a carbon cluster with a large mass similar to those he had found in interstellar matter. About a year later, Kroto received a favorable response to his request.

preliminary 予備の

As preparation for the joint research efforts proposed by Kroto, preliminary experiments using graphite plates were implemented on carbon clusters. At the time, a post-graduate researcher who was operating the mass spectroscope during these preliminary experiments noticed the existence of a strong peak in response to carbon-60. However, Kroto and his group failed to recognize this great discovery, as they were concentrating on clusters having a very small mass.

A similar missed opportunity had occurred at an Exxon research laboratory as well. Sumio Iijima of NEC (also a professor at Meijo University) who later discovered the carbon nanotube had observed an "onion-like globe" under an electron microscope in 1980 and had written a paper in which he noted that "twelve pentagons in addition to a hexagon are necessary." In short, Iijima had actually observed the new carbon structure C_{60}, but failed to recognize the importance of his discovery, while Smalley and his colleagues noticed the existence of C_{60} and gained the great honor of being credited with the discovery.

preconception 先入観, 偏見
novel 新規の, 今までにない

This episode tells us that even if there are some new discoveries in measured data, it is often very difficult to recognize them. Preconceptions must be eliminated first through the flow of new knowledge in order to make new discoveries. This is a lesson provided by the story behind the discovery of the fullerene—a truly novel substance.

出典: Naoki Ikezawa, "Nanotechnology: Encounters of Atoms, Bits and Genomes", NRI Papers, No. 37, p.8〜9 (2001)より許可を得て転載.

3. The Story Behind the Discovery of the Fullerene   17

3・2 Reading Comprehension

▶ **Question**   Answer the following questions in English.

対応 SBO
SBO 4

1. When did Smalley, Curl, and Kroto discover the existence of the fourth type of carbon molecule?

   _____

   _____

2. In the past, how many basic types of carbon molecules did scientists believe to exist?

   _____

   _____

3. Why didn't the book *Properties of Aromatics* attract considerable attention?

   _____

   _____

4. Why do scientists compete to name a new discovery?

   _____

   _____

5. To make new discoveries, what must be removed through the flow of new knowledge?

   _____

   _____

3・3 Grammatical Rule: 等位接続詞（Coordinate Conjunctions）

対応 SBO
SBOs 2,4,5

　両腕を左右に伸ばした母親に二人の子供がそれぞれの腕につかまっている様子を想像してみよう．等位接続詞とはちょうどその母親のようなものである．等位接続詞は，左右に同種の語句しか置けないという原則がある．したがって，右腕に大人，左腕に子供ということはタブーである．

　等位接続詞には and（そして，〜と〜），or（あるいは），nor（〜も〜ない），but（しかし，〜か〜），yet（しかし，けれども）などがある．

　では，本文中の下記の文の下線部には等位接続詞が使われている．何と何を左右に対等の関係で結びつけているか考えてみよう．and の右側を見ればヒントが見つかるだろう．

> At the time, Smalley and Curl had been searching for clusters with a specific molecular weight through a process of bombarding silicon and germanium with laser beams **and** analyzing the evaporating clusters (groups of atoms) by mass spectroscopy.

18   3. The Story Behind the Discovery of the Fullerene

対応 SBO
SBO 5

3・4 Writing

以下の作文をしなさい．

1. この大学では，1年生（first-year students）はドイツ語かフランス語か中国語を選択する（take）ことになっています．

   _____
   _____

2. 学食で A ランチを頼むと，主菜（main dish）にご飯，みそ汁，サラダがつきます．

   _____
   _____
   _____

3. アルバイトで帰宅が遅れたが，水曜日締切の宿題をなんとか終えた．

   _____
   _____
   _____

4. お天気が良くても悪くても（Rain or shine），バス停に 10 時に来るように，部員に伝えてください．

   _____
   _____
   _____

対応 SBO
SBOs 3,13

3・5 Medical Vocabulary

Write the name of each numbered part on the corresponding line.

(1) 大　脳　_____

(2) 小　脳　_____

(3) 視床下部　_____

(4) 下垂体　_____

(5) 脊　髄　_____

3・6 Listening/Speaking

▶ **Dictation** Listen to the following conversation and fill in the blanks.

対応 SBO
SBOs 10,12
Track 6

In a Hallway

Taro Yamada: Hi, my name is Taro. I (   ) yesterday's party Professor Nagai (   ) for you and Lisa. Can I ask you a question?
Bruce Chen: Hi. Sure, go ahead.
Taro Yamada: (   ) are you from?
Bruce Chen: I'm from Orange County, California. It's between L.A. and San Diego.
Taro Yamada: You're from the O.C.? (   ).
Bruce Chen: Have you been to the O.C.?
Taro Yamada: No, but I love the T.V. show. I have all of the DVDs.
Bruce Chen: That's (   ). I have never watched the show!
Taro Yamada: Really? It's one of my dreams to go to the O.C. one of these days.
Bruce Chen: Well, (   ). It's really nice.
Taro Yamada: Thanks, I hope so, too.

Now work with your partner and try to say the above dialog (in natural English).

Naturally Spoken English Notes:

that's so = thatsso   go to = goda

Chapter 4

Acid Rain

Objectives

After studying this chapter, you should be able to:
- Explain how acid rain is produced in Japanese or English. [SBO 2]
- Explain the content of English, including technical terms, related to pharmacy in English or Japanese. [SBO 3]
- Correctly explain English written for the sciences in Japanese or English. [SBO 4]
- Utilize one of the basic grammatical rules, adverbial to-infinitive, for reading and writing. [SBOs 2, 4, 5]
- List basic measurements, numbers, and phenomena related to the natural sciences. [SBO 7]
- Tell the difference between sounds in spoken English. [SBO 10]
- Correctly pronounce the names of medical equipment and subjects for pharmacy. [SBO 13]

対応 SBO

SBO 2

4・1 Reading

> 子どものころ，雨の中を走り回って遊んだことがある．それは愉快で楽しい思い出だが，いつごろからか雨に濡れると危ないという話を聞くようになった．空から降ってくる雨が人や物を傷つけてしまうほど酸性が強くなってしまったのはなぜだろう．ここでは，酸性雨の成り立ちと影響を化学的視点から考えてみよう．

Track 7

lightning 雷

Normally while rain travels through the air, it dissolves floating chemicals and washes down particles that are suspended in air. At the start of its journey raindrops are neutral (pH＝7). In clean air, rain picks up materials that occur naturally such as dust, pollen, some CO_2 and other chemicals produced by lightning or volcanic activities. These substances make rain slightly acidic (pH＝6), which is not dangerous. However, when rain falls through polluted air, it comes across chemicals such as gaseous oxides of sulphur (SO_x), oxides of nitrogen (NO_x), mists of acids such as hydrochloric and phosphoric acid, released from automobile exhausts, industrial plants, electric power plants etc.

These substances dissolve in falling rain making it more acidic than normal with a pH range between 5.6–3.5. In some cases, its pH gets lowered to the extent of 2. This leads to acid rain. The term acid rain is used here to describe all types of precipitation, namely, rain, snow, fog and dew more acidic than normal.

hydrochloric acid
塩酸
phosphoric acid
リン酸

Chemistry of Acid Rain

In the natural processes of volcanic eruptions, forest fires and bacterial decomposition of organic oxides of sulphur and nitrogen, production and reductions of gases naturally tend to an equilibrium. Power plants, smelting plants, industrial plants, burning of coal and automobile exhausts, release additional sulphur dioxide, nitrogen oxides and acidic soot, causing pollution. Sulphur dioxide and nitrogen dioxide interact with water vapours in the presence of sunlight to form sulphuric acid and nitric acid mist.

decomposition
分解, 腐敗
equilibrium　平衡
smelting plant
精錬工場

sulphuric acid　硫酸
nitric acid　硝酸

$$SO_2 + H_2O \longrightarrow H_2SO_3$$
Sulphurous acid

$$SO_2 + O_3 \longrightarrow SO_3 + O_2; \quad SO_3 + H_2O \longrightarrow H_2SO_4$$
Ozone　　　　　　　　　　　　　　　　　Sulphuric acid

$$2\,NO + O_2 \longrightarrow 2\,NO_2; \quad 2\,NO_2 + H_2O \longrightarrow HNO_3 + HNO_2$$
Nitric acid　Nitrous acid

The formed sulphuric acid and nitric acid remain as vapours at high temperatures. These begin to condense as the temperature falls and mix with rain or snow, on the way down to the Earth and make rain sufficiently acidic.

Harmful Effects of Acid Rain

SO_x, NO_x mixed with water as acid rain causes plant, animal and material damage. Some of the significant ill effects of acid rain are:

Damage to Animals

Acid rain chemically strips waterways of necessary nutrients and lowers the pH to levels where plants and animals cannot live. Most of the aquatic animals cannot survive when the pH is less than 4. Some species of fish, such as salmon, die even when the pH is less than 5.5. Certain species of algae and zooplankton are eliminated at a pH of less than 6. A reduction in the zooplankton and bottom fauna ultimately affects the food availability for the fish population. The problem is most severe downwind of industrial areas where fishing and tourism are major sources of income such as in Norway and Sweden.

Damage to Plants

Acidic water is dangerous to plants. Sulphuric and nitric acid rain washes nutrients out of the soil, damages the bark and leaves of trees and harms the fine root hairs of many plants which are needed to absorb water. Leaf pigments are decolorized because acid affects the green pigment (chlorophyll) of plants. Agricultural productivity is also decreased. Several non-woody plants, such as barley, cotton and fruit trees like apple, pear, etc., are severely affected by acid rain. Since the acid concentration increases near the base of clouds by density, high altitude trees and vegetation may be exposed to pH levels as low as 3. Unique areas such as the Black Forest in Germany and sugar maples in Vermont (USA) are particularly threatened.

Material Damage

Metallic surfaces exposed to acid rain are easily corroded. Textile fabrics, paper and leather products lose their material strength or disintegrate by acid rain. Building materials such as limestone, marble, dolomite, mortar and slate are weakened on reaction with acid rains because of the formation of soluble compounds.

$$CaCO_3 + H_2SO_4 \longrightarrow CaSO_4 + H_2O + CO_2$$

Thus, acid rain is dangerous for historical monuments.

disintegrate
崩壊する，分解する
dolomite　白雲石
slate　粘板石

出 典：©2010 TutorVista.com, http://www.tutorvista.com/content/chemistry/chemistry-iii/environmental-chemistry/acid-rain.php（2010 年 12 月 1 日現在）より許可を得て転載.

4・2　Reading Comprehension

▶ **Question**　A～J に入る最も適当なものを下から選べ.

Raindrops are (A) (pH=7) in clean air, picking up materials that occur (B). These substances make rain slightly (C) (pH=6), which is not dangerous. When rain falls (D) polluted air, it comes across chemicals and (E) of acids, released from (F) exhausts, industrial plants, electric (G) plants etc. Substances (H) in falling rain and make it more acidic than (I) with a pH range between 5.6–3.5. In some cases, its pH gets (J) to the extent of 2. This leads to acid rain.

対応 SBO
SBO 2

| acidic | automobile | dissolve | lowered | mists |
| naturally | neutral | normal | power | through |

4・3　Grammatical Rule：to 不定詞の副詞的用法
（**Adverbial To-infinitive**）

対応 SBO
SBOs 2,4,5

　to 不定詞の副詞的用法とは，文中の動詞，形容詞，副詞，文全体を修飾し，(1) 目的，(2) 原因・理由，(3) 仮定・条件，(4) 結果などの意味を表すもののことである．化学英語では，"結果"を表す不定詞用法がしばしば用いられ，ある現象・手順が先行し，"その結果～になる"というように訳すと意味がすっきりする場合が多くみられる．

　では，本文中の下記の例文を見てみよう．下線部が副詞的用法で"結果"を表していることを確認してみよう．

> Sulphur dioxide and nitrogen dioxide interact with water vapours in the presence of sunlight **to form sulphuric acid and nitric acid mist**.
> 　（二酸化硫黄と二酸化窒素は，太陽光線の存在下で水蒸気と相互作用を起こし，その結果，硫酸と硝酸の霧ができる．）

4・4 Writing

対応 SBO: SBO 7

数学に関する表現を練習しよう.

1. 英語で読みなさい.

   $y = x^4 + 9x^3 + kx$　_____

   $S = \dfrac{a}{b} + \dfrac{b}{a}$　_____

   $\cos^2 x + \sin^2 x = 1$　_____

2. 英語で答えなさい.

   (1) If you factor $x^2 - y^2$, what will you get?

   _____

   (2) If $a + 2b = 5$, what is the value of $3a$ and $6b$?

   _____

   (3) If $3x + y = 7$, what is x in terms of y?

   _____

4・5 Medical Vocabulary

対応 SBO: SBOs 3,13

Write the name of each numbered figure on the corresponding line.

(1) _____　(2) _____

(3) _____　(4) _____

(5) _____　(6) _____

(1) 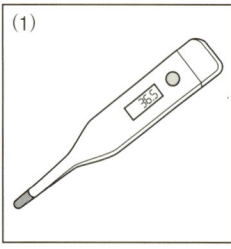　(2) 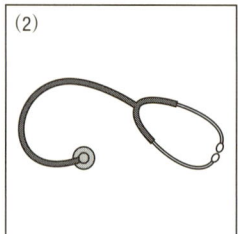　(3)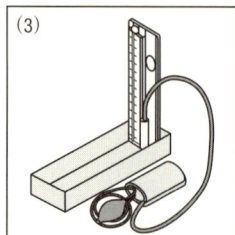

(4) 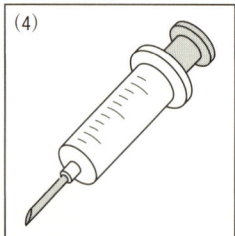　(5) 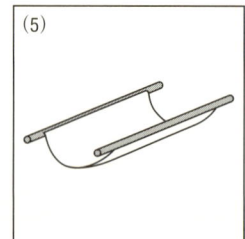　(6)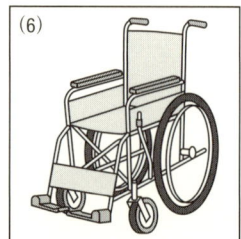

4・6 Listening/Speaking

▶ **Dictation**   Listen to the following conversation and fill in the blanks.

対応 SBO
SBOs 10,12,13
Track 8

At the University Library
Lisa Yamanaka：Yoko, hey, how are you?
Yoko Kimura：I'm OK, <u>but I</u> have a (   ) coming up and I really <u>have to</u> study.
Lisa Yamanaka：Which class is the test (   )?
Yoko Kimura：The test is on (   ) and I am not very good at it.
Lisa Yamanaka：I know <u>what you</u> mean! When I was studying the subject, I really (   ), too.
Yoko Kimura：Really? I thought you were so smart. I am sure you are very (   ) science.
Lisa Yamanaka：Actually, I'm not. I only studied to become a (   ) because of my parents.
Yoko Kimura：Really? I thought that was only in Japan! That's why I am here.
Lisa Yamanaka：No. We (   ). Anyway, good luck with your studies.
Yoko Kimura：Thanks. (   ).

Now work with your partner and try to say the above dialog (in natural English, of course), but use your own words. For example, instead of "organic chemistry," you could say, "anatomy."

Naturally Spoken English Notes：
but I = budai   have to = hafta   what you = whatcha
going to = gonna

Chapter 5

DNA

Objectives

After studying this chapter, you should be able to:

- Explain what DNA is in English or Japanese. [SBO 2]
- Describe in English or Japanese what the Human Genome Project is and how it will be utilized for genetic disorders. [SBO 2]
- Explain the content of English, including technical terms, related to pharmacy in Japanese or English. [SBO 3]
- Utilize one of the basic grammatical rules, gerunds, for reading and writing. [SBOs 2, 4, 5]
- List basic measurements, numbers, and phenomena related to the natural sciences in English or Japanese. [SBO 7]
- Outline the methods and results of a simple science experiment in English. [SBO 8]
- Tell the difference between sounds in spoken English. [SBO 10]
- Summarize the understood content of an English conversation between two pharmacy students. [SBO 11]
- Ask and answer questions that come up in an English conversation between two pharmacy students. [SBO 12]
- Correctly pronounce the names of illnesses and parts of the body. [SBO 13]

対応 SBO
SBO 2

5・1 Reading

自分はちっとも両親と似ていないと悩んだことはないだろうか．ところが気をつけて見てみると，髪の生え際の旋毛が父親そっくりだったり，足の指の形が母親そっくりだったりすることもある．病気の因子も例外ではない．ヒトの遺伝情報の解析が進み，そこから遺伝子治療への道が広がっている．一連の流れを科学的な視点からのぞいてみよう．

CD Track 9

chromosome 染色体
deoxyribonucleic acid デオキシリボ核酸

What Is DNA?

Chromosomes are X-shaped objects found in the nucleus of most cells. They consist of long strands of a substance called deoxyribonucleic acid, or DNA for short. A section of DNA that has the genetic code for making a particular protein is called a gene.

The gene is the unit of inheritance, and each chromosome may have several thousand genes. We inherit particular chromosomes through genes*. We inherit particular chromosomes through the egg of our mother and sperm of our father. The genes on those chromosomes carry the code that determines our physical characteristics, which are a combination of those of our two parents.

The bases in the DNA molecule carry the different codes needed for different amino acids. The code for a particular amino acid is made from three bases in a particular order.

Alleles and Genetic Disorders

Different forms of the same gene are called alleles. You inherit one allele for each gene from your father and one allele for each gene from your mother. For example, the gene for eye colour has an allele for blue eye colour and an allele for brown eye colour. Your eye colour will depend on the combination of alleles you have inherited from your parents.

Diseases can be caused by a number of things, including:

    infections   e.g. influenza
    poor diet   e.g. scurvy
    environmental factors   e.g. asbestosis
    spontaneous degeneration of tissues   e.g. multiple sclerosis

People with cystic fibrosis have inherited two faulty alleles, one from their father and one from their mother. They produce unusually thick and sticky mucus in their lungs and airways. Their lungs become congested with mucus, and they are more likely to get respiratory infections. Daily physiotherapy helps to relieve congestion, while antibiotics are used to fight infection. The disorder also affects the gut and pancreas, so that food is not digested efficiently.

The Human Genome Project

genome
ゲノム，全遺伝情報

The genetic information in an organism is called its genome. The Human Genome Project, or HGP for short, was started at the end of the last century. It was very ambitious and had several aims, including:

sequence 配列

- to work out the order or sequence of all the three billion base pairs in the human genome
- to identify all the genes
- to develop faster methods for sequencing DNA

The sequencing project was finished in 2001, and work continues to identify all the genes in the human genome. The HGP used the DNA of several people to get a sort of average sequence, but each person has a unique sequence (unless they have an identical twin).

Genetic Treatment of Disease

It is hoped that information from the Human Genome Project will allow scientists to develop new ways of treating or diagnosing illness, especially genetic disorders and cancer.

diagnose 診断する

A person with cystic fibrosis has inherited two faulty alleles for a certain gene on one of their chromosomes, chromosome 7. It is hoped that it may one day be possible to repair the faulty alleles using gene therapy, perhaps by putting the normal allele into the cells of the lungs. This would greatly improve the lives of people with cystic fibrosis, who often need a lung transplant as their illness progresses.

Members of some families are particularly at risk of developing certain types of breast cancer, because they carry faulty alleles. These alleles have been identified, and it is now possible to test people to see if they have an increased risk of developing breast cancer. This allows them to make decisions, if they wish, about whether to have surgery to remove breast tissue before any cancer develops in their breasts.

出 典：©BBC, http://www.bbc.co.uk/schools/gcsebitesize/science/edexcel/genes/dnarev_print.shtml（2010 年 12 月 1 日現在）より許可を得て転載．

5・2 Reading Comprehension

▶ **Question**　Answer the following questions in English.

1. What do chromosomes consist of？

2. What is the unit of inheritance called？

3. What are alleles？

4. How many faulty alleles has a person with cystic fibrosis inherited from his or her parents？

5. What aims did the Human Genome Project have？

6. What will the HGP help scientists to do in the field of medicine？

5・3 Grammatical Rule：動名詞（Gerunds）

　動名詞とは，"動詞＋-ing" と動詞に類似した形をとりながら，文中で名詞と同様の働きをするもののことである．つまり，文中の主語（S），補語（C），目的語（O），前置詞の目的語（prep. ＋O）として使われる．自然科学の英文では，前置詞の目的語として用いられることが多い．

　たとえば，"in binding ～：～を結合する際に"，"for identifying ～：～を同定するために"，"by replacing ～：～を置換することによって" などである．

　では，本文中の例文を見てみよう．下線部が動名詞句である．なぜ動名詞といえるのか考えてみよう．

> It is hopred that it may one day be possible to repair the faulty alleles using gene therapy, perhaps by <u>putting the normal allele into the cells of the lungs</u>.

30 5. DNA

対応 SBO
SBOs 7,8

5・4 Writing

化学変化に関する表現 —— 結果を表す to 不定詞

1. 英語にしなさい．

(1) 水素と酸素が反応して水ができる．($2H_2 + O_2 \longrightarrow 2H_2O$)

_____

_____

(2) マグネシウムと酸素が反応すると酸化マグネシウムができる．
($2Mg + O_2 \longrightarrow 2MgO$)

_____

_____

2. 英語で答え，化学反応式（chemical equation）を書きなさい．

(1) What happens when zinc reacts with hydrochloric acid?

_____

_____

(2) What happens when sodium oxide reacts with water?

_____

_____

_____

対応 SBO
SBOs 3,13

5・5 Medical Vocabulary

Write the name of each numbered part on the corresponding line.

上大静脈 superior vena cava
肺動脈弁 pulmonary valve
下大静脈 inferior vena cava
左心房 left atrium
左心室 left ventricle
心筋 myocardium
大動脈弁 aortic valve

(1) 右心房 _____
(2) 右心室 _____
(3) 大動脈 _____
(4) 肺動脈 _____
(5) 肺静脈 _____

5・6 Listening/Speaking

▶ **Dictation**   Listen to the following conversation and fill in the blanks.

対応 SBO
SBOs 10,11,12,13
CD Track 10

In the Lab
Lisa Yamanaka: Hey Bruce, can you (   )?
Bruce Chen: Sure, Lisa, what's wrong?
Lisa Yamanaka: I am trying to write a report about our stay here in Japan, but my
               computer won't start up.
Bruce Chen: Here, let me (   ). Hmmm...everything
               looks fine to me.
Lisa Yamanaka: It was working yesterday, but now it won't cooperate.
Bruce Chen: Well, while I try some things, (   )?
Lisa Yamanaka: Can I? That would be so nice of you. I really want to write up some
               of my notes on (   ) in hospitals in Japan.
Bruce Chen: Sure. And what did you find out?
Lisa Yamanaka: It's been very interesting, but a challenge. There isn't (
) like in the States.
Bruce Chen: Well, maybe Prof. Nagai can give you some suggestions. We'll (
) later.

Now work with your partner and try to say the above dialog (in natural English).

Naturally Spoken English Notes:

give me = gimme   computer = compuda   information = info
later = lader

COLUMN

海底温泉の生き物からわかったこと

1970年代後半までは，地球上の生命はすべて日光から光エネルギーを得ているという見方が優勢であった．1977年，二人の地質学者が水深2500mの深海にあるガラパゴスの海底火山の裂け目から熱水が噴出している一種の海底温泉のような場所で驚くべき発見をした．その熱水噴出孔からは，鉄（Fe），銅（Cu），亜鉛（Zn）などの金属元素と硫化水素（H_2S），水素（H_2），メタン（CH_4）などを含む熱水が噴出し，その周辺にワムシとよばれる水中の微小動物や二枚貝類，イソギンチャク，体が真っ白なエビ・カニの仲間などのさまざまな生物がびっしりと群集していたのである．ある種のミネラルから化学エネルギーを抽出し，硫化水素やメタンなどを材料に有機物を合成する化学合成過程を通して細菌が誕生し，この化学合成細菌を基礎生産者とした食物連鎖により化学合成生態系が成立したと考えられている．これまでは，太陽こそ，地球の生命を支えるエネルギーの源であるという概念が支配していたが，熱水噴出孔にいる生き物たちは，生命の多様性と能力に関する従来の仮説に再考を促すものとなった．

（市川　厚）

Chapter 6

The Nobel Prize in Chemistry (2001)

Objectives

After studying this chapter, you should be able to:

- Read simple written sentences and identify the main idea in a timely fashion.
  [SBO 1]
- Explain the content of simple written passages in Japanese or English. [SBO 2]
- Explain the study of the Nobel Prize in Chemistry (2001) in English or Japanese.
  [SBO 3]
- Correctly explain English written for the sciences and related to clinical practice in Japanese or English. [SBO 4]
- Utilize one of the basic grammatical rules, emphasis, for reading and writing.
  [SBOs 2, 4, 5]
- Rewrite short Japanese sentences into English without grammatical errors.
  [SBO 5]
- Outline the methods and results of a simple science experiment in English.
  [SBO 8]
- Write a simple paragraph related to the sciences or clinical practice in English.
  [SBO 9]
- Tell the difference between sounds in spoken English. [SBO 10]
- Correctly pronounce the names of illnesses, parts of the body, and drugs.
  [SBO 13]

対応 SBO
SBOs 1,2,3,4

6・1 Reading

ここで取上げられているのは，2001年，野依良治博士が William S. Knowles 博士，Barry K. Sharpless 博士とともにノーベル化学賞を受賞した際に，その業績が一般の人向けに紹介された記事である．研究内容をどのようにわかりやすく解説してあるだろうか．また，研究の社会的な意義についてどのように書かれているかにも留意しながら読もう．

CD Track 11

Mirror Image Catalysis

Chiral Molecules

This year's Nobel Prize in Chemistry concerns the way in which certain chiral molecules can be used to speed up and control important chemical reactions. The word *chiral* comes from the Greek word *cheir*, which means hand. Our hands are chiral—our right hand is a mirror image of our left hand—as are most of life's molecules. If, for example, we study the common amino acid alanine (Figure 1), we see that it can occur in two forms: (S)-alanine and (R)-alanine, which are mirror images.

(S)-alanine   mirror plane (R)-alanine

Figure 1 Chirality in the amino acid alanine is illustrated with models of its two forms, which are mirror images of each other. They are designated (S) and (R).

However we twist or turn these forms, we cannot get them to overlap each other. Apparently, they do not have the same three-dimensional structure. The reason is that the carbon atom in the centre binds the four different groups H, CH_3, NH_2 and COOH, which are located at the corners of a tetrahedron. The unbroken bonds to NH_2 and COOH indicate that these bonds are in the plane of the paper, whereas the black wedge shaped bond and the broken wedge shaped bond show that they are directed upwards and downwards respectively in relation to the plane of the paper.

tetrahedron 四面体

Thus the amino acid alanine occurs in two forms, called *enantiomers*. When alanine is produced in a laboratory under normal conditions, a mixture is obtained, half of which is (S)-alanine and the other (R)-alanine. The synthesis is symmetrical in the sense that it produces equal amounts of both enantiomers.

enantiomer 光学異性体, エナンチオマー

Asymmetric synthesis, on the other hand, deals with the production of an excess of one of the forms. Why is this so important? Let us go back to nature to find the answer.

asymmetric synthesis 不斉合成

Drugs and the Smell of Lemons

Most drugs consist of chiral molecules. And since a drug must match the molecules it should bind to itself in the cells, it is often only one of the enantiomers that is of interest. In certain cases, the other form may even be harmful. This was the case, for example, with the drug thalidomide, which was sold in the 1960s to pregnant women. One of the enantiomers of thalidomide helped against nausea, while the other one could cause foetal damage.

There are other, less dramatic examples of how differently the two enantiomers can affect our cells. Limonene, for example, is chiral, but the two enantiomers can be difficult to distinguish at first glance (Figure 2). The receptors in our nose are more sensitive. One form certainly smells of lemons but the other of oranges.

(R)-limonene   mirror plane   (S)-limonene

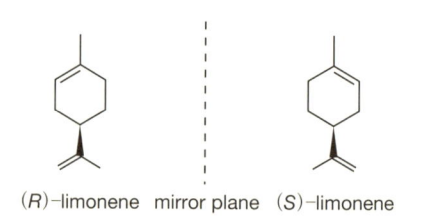

Figure 2 (R)-limonene smells of oranges while its enantiomer (S)-limonene smells of lemons

Catalytic Asymmetric Synthesis—What Is It?

It is very important for industry to be able to produce products as pure as possible. It is also important to be able to manufacture large quantities of a product. For this reason the use of catalysts is very important. A catalyst is a substance that increases the rate of the reaction without being consumed itself.

During the past few decades there has been intensive research into developing methods for producing—synthesising—one of the enantiomers rather than the other. In a synthesis, starting molecules (substrate molecules) are used to build new molecules (products) by means of various chemical reactions. It is to researchers in this field that this year's Nobel Prize in Chemistry has been awarded. The Laureates have developed chiral catalysts for two important classes of reactions in organic chemistry: hydrogenations and oxidations.

substrate molecule
基質分子

laureate 受賞者

hydrogenation
水素化，水素添加

出典：©The Royal Swedish Academy of Sciences, http://www.kva.se/Documents/Priser/Nobel/2001/pop_ke_en_01.pdf（2010年12月1日現在）より許可を得て転載．

6・2 Reading Comprehension

The following is a summary of the passage. Fill the gaps with words from the passage. Change the form of the words when necessary.

対応 SBO
SBOs 8,9

1. The word chiral has its origin in the (　　　) word *cheir*, and it means (　　　). Chiral forms cannot (　　　) no matter how they are twisted or (　　　).

2. In the production of alanine in a laboratory, two (　　　) can be obtained and each amount is about the same. Therefore, this type of synthesis is called (　　　) synthesis.

3. The drug thalidomide is an (　　　) of the enantiomers which turned out to have utterly different effects.

4. (*R*)-limonene and (*S*)-limonene may look similar but can be (　　　) by their (　　　).

5. In 2001, scientists were (　　　) the Nobel Prize in Chemistry, because they succeeded in (　　　) chiral catalysts for hydrogenations and (　　　).

6・3 Grammatical Rule：強調（Emphasis）

ある語句を強調するための方法にはどのようなものがあるか，思い出してみよう．

対応 SBO
SBOs 2,4,5

(1) 倒置による強調
　　Not a word did she say about my proposal.
(2) It is ～ that (who, which など) …による強調
　　It is you **who** are to blame.
(3) 助動詞 do による強調
　　He said he would work hard, and actually he **did** study six hours every day.
(4) 修辞疑問による強調
　　Who knows my real feelings?（= Nobody knows my real feelings.）

(5) 反復による強調

　　The patient came to the pharmacy **again and again**.

(6) 強意の語句を用いた強調

　　The lecture was **not at all** enjoyable.

では，次の例文は，どのような意味になるか考えてみよう．

> But **it was** *not until the 1980's* **that** we understood the cause of the problem.

6・4 Writing

元素記号と比較表現

Table 1   Examples of Relative Atomic Mass

Symbol	Relative Atomic Mass	Symbol	Relative Atomic Mass
C	12.01	O	16.00
H	1.01	Fe	55.85
He	4.00	Cu	63.55
N	14.01		

1. この表に合うように，カッコ内に適当な単語を入れなさい．

   (1) Carbon atoms are (　　　　) times heavier than hydrogen atoms.

   (2) The mass of copper atoms is approximately (　　　　) times bigger than that of oxygen atoms.

2. これに倣って二つの元素記号を選びそれらを比較する文を2文つくりなさい．

   (1) _____

   (2) _____

6・5 Medical Vocabulary

Write the name of each numbered part on the corresponding line.

(1) 腎盂（じんう）　_____

(2) 腎臓　_____

(3) 尿管　_____

(4) 膀胱　_____

(5) 尿道　_____

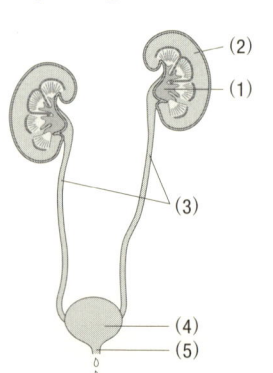

6·6 Listening/Speaking

▶ **Dictation** Listen to the following conversation and fill in the blanks.

対応 SBO
SBO 10
Track 12

In the Lab

Prof. Nagai: Knock, knock. It's almost six o'clock. (　　　　　)?

Bruce and Lisa: Hey Prof. Nagai. Sure. What should we do for dinner?

Prof. Nagai: Well, my students and I were going to get some pizza. Would you like (　　　　　)?

Lisa Yamanaka: Ooh, I heard about pizza in Japan. (　　　　　)!

Bruce Chen: You mean the pizza (　　　　　)?

Prof. Nagai: Yes, we have all kinds. We get very creative with our pizza.

Lisa Yamanaka: I am so happy I brought my camera with me. I am going to put the pictures on my Facebook account.

Prof. Nagai: You know many of my students also like (　　　　　), especially sweets.

Lisa Yamanaka: Well, I am sure (　　　　　) will love the pictures.

Prof. Nagai: I'm sure they will. The Internet has (　　　　　) helped make the world smaller.

Now work with your partner and try to say the above dialog (in natural English), but use your own words. For example, instead of "squid" or "octopus" think of other pizza toppings.

Naturally Spoken English Notes:

octopus = acdapus　　yes = yep　　pictures = pics

COLUMN

アミノ酸とペプチド

アミノ酸は分子内にアミノ基（-NH$_2$）とカルボキシ基（-COOH）の二つの官能基が存在している化合物をいうが，薬学の分野ではカルボキシ基が結合しているα位の炭素原子にアミノ基も結合しているアミノ酸 R-CH(NH$_2$)-COOH のことをさすのが一般的である．生体に存在しているアミノ酸は一般にL形（Lは S, R 同様立体構造を表す記号．逆の立体はDと表記する．）の構造をとっていて，栄養源となる．Rを側鎖とよび，Rの異なる20種類のアミノ酸が生体内に存在している．

アミノ基とカルボキシ基とが分子間で脱水縮合して連なった化合物〔-NH(R-CH)-CO-〕$_n$ がペプチドで，その結合をペプチド結合という．多数のペプチド結合から成る高分子がポリペプチドで，分子量1万以上のポリペプチドがタンパク質である．

タンパク質は私たちの生命活動に不可欠な物質で，身体の基本骨格の形成，生化学反応の触媒（酵素），栄養物質の運搬（輸送）など多様な役割を担っている．タンパク質の機能は構成しているアミノ酸残基Rにより決定される．Rがどのような機能に関係しているかを知ることは非常に大切である．

（寺田 弘）

Chapter 7

The Race to Synthesize Taxol

Objectives

After studying this chapter, you should be able to:
- Explain the content of simple written passages in Japanese or English.　　[SBO 2]
- Explain in Japanese and English what kind of drug Taxol is and how it is made.
　　　　　　　　　　　　　　　　　　　　　　　　　　　　　　　　　[SBO 3]
- Correctly explain English written for the sciences in Japanese or English.　[SBO 4]
- Utilize one of the basic grammatical rules, five sentence patterns, for reading and writing.　　　　　　　　　　　　　　　　　　　　　　　　　　[SBOs 2, 4, 5]
- Rewrite short Japanese sentences about Japanese culture and campus life into English without grammatical errors.　　　　　　　　　　　　　　　　[SBO 5]
- Outline the methods and results of a simple science experiment in English.[SBO 8]
- Explain the content of English, including technical terms, related to pharmacy in Japanese or English.　　　　　　　　　　　　　　　　　　　　　　　[SBO 3]
- Tell the difference between sounds in spoken English.　　　　　　　　[SBO 10]
- Correctly pronounce parts of the body.　　　　　　　　　　　　　　[SBO 13]

対応 SBO
SBOs 2,3,4

7・1 Reading

> Taxol は抗癌剤として臨床で使われており薬剤師にとって重要な薬剤である．タキサン系抗癌剤の年間総売上高は 3,000 億円を超える．天然からの供給量に限りがあるため有機合成法の確立が望まれていた．しかし，taxol の構造は複雑であり効率的な合成法の確立は困難を極めた．世界中の名だたる研究者が競った末，構造決定から 20 年以上の歳月を経て 1994 年にその合成法が報告された．ぜひ原著にもふれてみよう．

CD Track 13

"Devising a total synthesis of the anti-cancer drug taxol has engaged the attention of chemists for more than 20 years. But their ingenuity—and perseverance—has been rewarded". Thus the journal *Nature* on 17 February 1994 announced the first published total synthesis of taxol by K.C. Nicolaou and his group at the Scripps Research Institute in California[1]. Within a week, Bob Holton and his group at Florida State

total synthesis　全合成：安価で入手しやすい出発物質から目的とする天然有機化合物を合成すること．

University also published a total synthesis of taxol[2]. The journal *Chemistry and Industry* described the two events as a "photo-finish in the race to artificial taxol".

artificial 人工の

Taxol

The various approaches to developing methods of obtaining taxol that we have so far discussed all depended on harnessing biological processes. These included extraction from bark or renewable parts of various *Taxus* species, extraction from *Taxomyces* fungus, extraction from *Taxus* cell culture; and semi-synthesis from taxanes related structurally to taxol and from *Taxus* species that can be cultivated. In contrast to all these, total synthesis uses chemical processes to make taxol from inexpensive starting materials—including naturally-occurring ones—and has nothing to do with yew trees at all.

It was automatic for chemists to try and make taxol by total synthesis as soon as its structure was known. Total synthesis harnesses the specific skills of organic chemists, and represents a major challenge to their chemical ingenuity: "conquering a molecular Mount Everest". Tackling the problems of synthesis also generates chemical knowledge about structure, reactions, properties, mechanisms of action, and new approaches to synthesis. Moreover, during the process of exploring the synthetic alternatives, analogues are likely to be produced that are potentially simpler and medicinally more effective, or have improved properties (more soluble, or less toxic for instance). Some chemists are also attracted by the aesthetic as well as scientific appeal of complex

harnessing 利用
extraction 抽出
bark 樹皮
Taxus species イチイ種
Taxomyces fungus *Taxomyces* 菌
semi-synthesis 半合成：天然から入手可能な化合物を出発原料としてそれを修飾することで目的物を合成すること．
cultivate 培養する
yew trees イチイの木

synthetic alternatives 合成代替品
analogues 類似化合物，類縁体，アナログ：ある物質の一部の原子あるいは置換基などの部分構造を化学変換した類似物質をさす．薬剤のアナログは薬物動態の調節や新たな薬理活性の付与が期待され有用である．

* 標的化合物を複数のパーツに分け、これらを連結することにより合成を行う際、これらのパーツのことをビルディングブロックとよぶ。

molecules: the way in which the building blocks* of taxol's architecture, for example, are represented by 112 atoms arranged in space.

As we have seen, several groups of chemists began work on taxol in the early 1980s, including Charles Swindell at Bryn Mawr College, Bob Holton at Virginia Polytechnic Institute (later at Florida State University), David Kingston at Virginia Polytechnic Institute, Paul Wender at Stanford University, and Pierre Potier at the institute de Chimie des Substances Naturelles. All but Potier were primarily interested in total synthesis. Chemists were therefore working on the total synthesis of taxol long before the supply problems had been defined and, with the exception of Potier's group, generally before the work began on semi-synthesis. The earlier work was not aiming at a practical, commercializable route, but was an exercise in developing chemical knowledge. According to Paul Wender, "we defined the problems initially as...requiring the development of a new synthetic methodology...It was a fundamental problem (and) if we were successful...we would put back into the synthetic chemist's box of tools some significant new tools that will be useful for problems that... show up in the future".

clinical trials　治験

Once the clinical trials of taxol revealed the seriousness of the supply problem, the largely academic approach to total synthesis in the United States gave way to a more practical concern.

From the point of view of the supply problem, if total synthesis were to provide a solution it would have had to be a "practical" synthesis: that is, one which could be scaled-up from laboratory to industrial preparation, and one which was comparable in cost with existing processes, or cheaper.

preparation　合成

出　典："The Story of Taxol" p.176〜178 (2001), ⓒJordan Goodman, Vivien Walsh, published by Cambridge University Press より許可を得て転載.

参考文献： 1) Nicolaou, K. C. *et al. Nature*, **1994**, *367*, 630.
　　　　　 2) Holton, R. A. *et al. J. Am. Chem. Soc.*, **1994**, *116*, 1597, 1599.

7. The Race to Synthesize Taxol

7・2 Reading Comprehension

▶ **Question**　Answer each question in English.

対応 SBO
SBOs 2,3,4,8

1. What kind of drug is Taxol?
　_____

2. What does "photo-finish in the race to artificial taxol" in the first paragraph mean?
　_____

3. What is the merit of total synthesis using chemical processes in contrast to biological processes?
　_____

4. What does "conquering a molecular Mount Everest" mean?
　_____

5. What does "practical synthesis" in the last paragraph mean?
　_____

7・3　Grammatical Rule：5文型（Five Sentence Patterns）

対応 SBO
SBOs 2,4,5

英語の文を五つに分類することは，元来，無理であるが，動詞の種類によって，伝統的に5文型に分ける考え方がある．ここで再確認してみよう．

　第1文型　　主語＋自動詞（S＋V）

　第2文型　　主語＋自動詞＋補語（S＋V＋C）　　S＝Cの意味関係が成立．

　第3文型　　主語＋他動詞＋目的語（S＋V＋O）　　S≠Oである．

　第4文型　　主語＋他動詞＋間接目的語＋直接目的語（S＋V＋IO＋DO）

　第5文型　　主語＋他動詞＋目的語＋補語（S＋V＋O＋C）
　　　　　　　　O＝Cの意味関係が成立．

動詞の種類は自動詞と他動詞に分けられ，目的語をとる動詞を他動詞，それ以外を自動詞とよぶ．自然科学の英文には第3文型が最も頻繁に用いられている．本文の第一段落は，まさに第3文型の連続であることに気づいただろうか．

では，本文中の次の文は何文型か考えてみよう．

　These included extraction from bark or renewable parts of various *Taxus* species, extraction from *Taxomyces* fungus, extraction from *Taxus* cell culture; and semi-synthesis from taxanes related structurally to taxol and from *Taxus* species that can be cultivated.

7. The Race to Synthesize Taxol

対応 SBO
SBO 5

7・4 Writing

折れ線グラフ（Line Graph）の読み方を学ぼう．

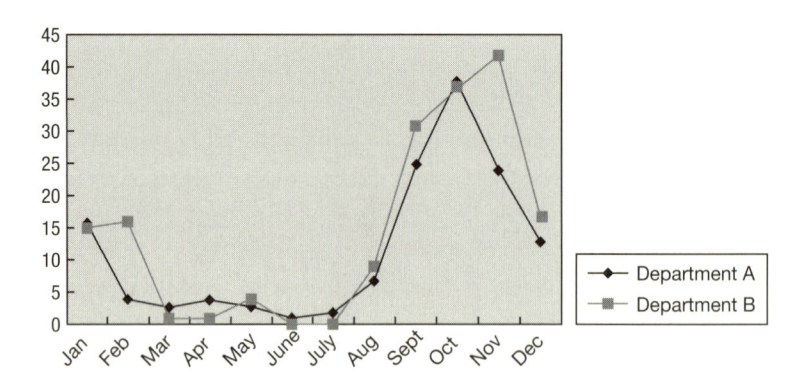

Number of Influenza Cases Reported at ABC University in 2009

この表からどのようなことが言えるだろうか．

例：(1) The number of cases for both departments increased dramatically from August to September.

(2) Department B had few cases from March to July.

例に倣って，図から言えることを二つあげなさい．必要ならばまず日本語でアイディアを出したり，友人と相談したりしてもよい．

_____

_____

_____

対応 SBO
SBOs 3,13

7・5 Medical Vocabulary

Write the name of each numbered part on the corresponding line.

(1) 外　耳　_____　(2) 外耳道　_____

(3) 鼓　膜　_____　(4) 蝸　牛　_____

(5) 中　耳　_____

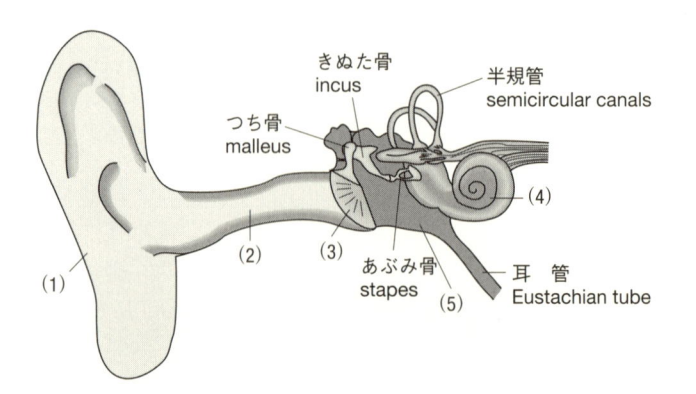

7・6 Listening/Speaking

▶ **Dictation**   Listen to the following conversation and fill in the blanks.

At a Train Station near the University
Taro Yamada：Hello Bruce. What are you doing?
Bruce Chen：I am looking at (　　　　　　　　　　). I really want to go to Akihabara.
Taro Yamada：Well, as a matter of fact, I am going to go shopping there tomorrow. (　　　　　　　　　) to go with me?
Bruce Chen：That would be great! I haven't really used the trains so much and am a little worried (　　　　　　　).
Taro Yamada：No worries. I am glad (　　　　　　　　　).
Bruce Chen：So, (　　　　　　　) should I meet you tomorrow?
Taro Yamada：How about at the main entrance of the university?
Bruce Chen：(　　　　　　　　). And what time?
Taro Yamada：(　　　　　　　　　). If we meet then, we'll arrive at Akihabara before noon.
Bruce Chen：All right. See you then.

Now work with your partner and try to say the above dialog (in natural English), but use your own words. For example, instead of "Akihabara," you could say, "Shinjuku." And instead of "main entrance," you could say, "library."

Naturally Spoken English Notes：

what are ＝ whad're　　a matter of fact ＝ amadderafact
tomorrow ＝ tamorrow　　little ＝ liddle　　university ＝ universidy

---

COLUMN

せっかち，それとも，ゆったり

　有機合成化学の研究者や技術者にはせっかちな人が多い．せっかちが幸いして研究が上手く進むこともあれば，災いして残念な結果で終わることもある．とある日，その有機合成化学の教授は，大学院生の実験が遅いのに業を煮やして自分で反応を薄層クロマトグラフィーでモニターすることにした．反応開始後2時間で原料スポットが消えたので，しめしめ私がやったから上手くいったぞと喜び，反応を止めて生成物の構造を確認した．しかし期待した**1**と**2**ではなく，**3**が生成物だったのでがっくり．しかし翌日，同じ反応をやっていた修士課程の院生が，"先生，上手くいきました，最初に**3**が確認できましたが，続けるとしだいに**1**と**2**に平衡がずれました．速度論生成物の**3**が熱力学生成物**1**と**2**に移行したんです．一晩ゆっくり反応させるのが成功のもとです"と報告した．

(富岡 清)

Chapter 8

Copper

Objectives

After studying this chapter, you should be able to:

- Read simple written sentences and identify the main idea in a timely fashion. [SBO 1]
- Explain the content of simple written passages in Japanese or English. [SBO 2]
- Explain in English or Japanese how copper works in our body. [SBO 3]
- Correctly explain English written for the sciences and related to clinical practice in Japanese or English. [SBO 4]
- Utilize one of the basic grammatical rules, subjunctive present, for reading and writing. [SBOs 2, 4, 5]
- Rewrite short Japanese sentences about Japanese culture and campus life into English without grammatical errors. [SBO 5]
- Outline the results of a simple graph in English. [SBO 8]
- Write a simple paragraph related to the sciences or clinical practice in English. [SBO 9]
- Tell the difference between sounds in spoken English. [SBO 10]
- Correctly pronounce the names of illnesses, parts of the body, and cells. [SBO 13]

対応 SBO
SBOs 1,2,3,4

8・1 Reading

銅イオンは生体内で機能する代表的な金属イオンの一つである．一方，銅は毒性の強い元素であり，社会的，歴史的には足尾銅山鉱毒事件，瀬戸内海の直島銅精錬所などの公害問題をひき起こした．また現代ではサプリメントに含まれることがあり，過剰摂取が懸念されている．銅が生体内反応でどのような役割を担っているかを理解しよう．

CD
Track 15

bran　ふすま
lentil　ヒラマメ

gut　消化器官

Copper is a required nutrient. It is found naturally in foods such as seafood, liver, green vegetables, whole grains, wheat bran, lentils, and nuts. Copper helps regulate blood pressure and heart rate and is needed to absorb iron from the gut. It is used to make many important compounds in the body.

Overview

Some laboratory and animal studies have found that copper has antioxidant properties and may have some anti-cancer effects. Other studies have found that high copper levels in the blood were linked with cancer and other diseases. More extensive human studies are needed to determine what role copper may play in the prevention or treatment of cancer.

How Is It Promoted for Use?

There are claims that copper aids in the healing process, helps to expel toxins from the body, and helps prevent heart problems. Copper is also used in some preparations of Iscador, a commercially prepared mistletoe extract sold as a complementary therapy in Europe for tumors of the liver, gallbladder, stomach, and kidneys.

There are also claims that copper actually promotes cancer growth. Proponents of this theory recommend a diet low in copper and the use of chelating agents that bind to copper and promote its elimination from the body.

What Does It Involve?

Copper supplements are available in pill or capsule form. Copper is often added to vitamin supplements. However, most people are able to get enough copper in their bodies by eating balanced meals. Fruits and vegetables can provide up to 30% of a person's total copper intake. Some copper is also present in drinking water, and copper pipes can leach extra copper into the water they carry.

The minimum recommended dietary allowance (RDA) for copper is 0.9 milligrams per day for most adults, 1 milligram for pregnant women, and 1.3 milligrams for women who are breast-feeding. The RDA is enough to meet the needs of most people in these groups.

What Is the History Behind It?

While research into the antioxidant properties of copper is quite recent, healing properties have long been attributed to copper in folk medicine. Some people wear copper bracelets, for example, to help with arthritis. Today, many multivitamins and other herbal and mineral supplements include copper.

What Is the Evidence?

Copper is a trace mineral that is needed for many important body processes. Animal studies have shown that copper is useful in maintaining antioxidant defenses. Antioxidants block the actions of free radicals, activated oxygen molecules that can damage cells. While the role of copper in the cancer process is still unclear, copper complexes have been shown to have anti-cancer properties in laboratory studies.

Other laboratory and animal studies suggest that high copper levels may be linked to liver cancer and brain tumors. More recently, many studies have shown that patients' blood copper levels are higher in several types of cancer and other diseases. To add to the confusion, blood tests can show high copper levels even when there is little copper in the tissues. These high copper levels may be due to injury, disease, or inflammation.

Because copper is needed to form new blood vessels, and because cancer needs new blood vessels in order to grow, some researchers are interested in copper's possible impact on cancer. One group of researchers looked at whether a copper-lowering drug could help patients with advanced kidney cancer. Some patients' cancer stopped growing during the 6-month treatment period. A few people had low white blood counts during treatment, requiring that treatment be stopped until they recovered. This was a small study, and further research is needed to find out whether copper can help more people with advanced cancer.

出 典： Reprint by the permission of the American Cancer Society, Inc. from www.cancer.org. All rights reserved.

8・2 Reading Comprehension

対応 SBO
SBOs 1,2,4,9

▶ **Question**   Answer the following questions in English.

1. What kinds of food include copper?
   _____

2. According to some laboratory and animal studies, what properties does copper have?
   _____

3. What kind of drug is Iscador?
   _____

4. How much copper per day should pregnant women take at a minimum?
   _____

5. According to animal studies, how is copper useful?
   _____

8・3 Grammatical Rule：仮定法現在（Subjunctive Present）

対応 SBO
SBOs 2,4,5

英語の法（mood）には直説法と仮定法がある．直説法は事実を述べる際に用いる一般的な用法である．これに対し，"主語が何であれ動詞の原形を用い，時制の一致に左右されず，話者の心の中で想定された事柄を表すもの" を仮定法現在という．
仮定法現在が使われる条件は，以下のような場合である．

（1） 提案・勧告・要求・主張・命令・決定などを表す動詞に続く that 節の中（advise, ask, demand, determine, insist, propose, recommend, request, require, suggest など，および，これらの動詞から派生した形容詞，名詞の後の that 節中）
   I suggested that we **not come** to the conclusion so soon.

（2） It is necessary that ... などの that 節中（advisable, anxious, desirable, essential, important, necessary, proper など）
   It is necessary that she **see** a doctor at once.

では，下記の本文中の例文で用いられている仮定法現在は，話者のどのような心情を表しているか考えてみよう．

> A few people had low white blood counts during treatment, requiring **that treatment be stopped** until they recovered.

8. Copper

対応 SBO
SBOs 5,8

8・4 Writing

棒グラフ（Bar Graph）の読み方を学ぼう．

例：(1) In 2008, there were three times as many undergraduates with the measles as in 2004.
(2) In 2000, no graduate students were infected with the measles.

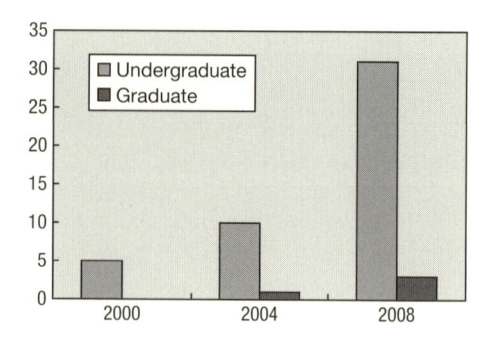

Number of Cases of Measles Reported at ABC University

1. グラフから言えることを二つあげなさい．必要ならばまず日本語でアイディアを出したり，友人と相談したりしてもよい．

_____

_____

_____

2. この表から，あなたが学部長であればどのような対策をとるか．文を完成させなさい．

   If I were the dean of ABC University, ～

_____

_____

対応 SBO
SBO 13

8・5 Medical Vocabulary

Write the name of each numbered part on the corresponding line.

(1) 原形質膜　　_____

(2) 核　　_____

(3) リソソーム　　_____

(4) ゴルジ装置　　_____

(5) ミトコンドリア

　　_____

図中ラベル：
- 中心小体 centriole
- 核小体 nucleolus
- 粗面小胞体 rough endoplasmic reticulum (ER)
- 核膜 nuclear membrane
- 細胞質ゾル cytosol
- 滑面小胞体 smooth endoplasmic reticulum (ER)
- リボソーム ribosome

8·6 Listening/Speaking

▶ **Dictation** Listen to the following conversation and fill in the blanks.

In a Lecture Hall

Lisa Yamanaka: Yoko, (   )?
Yoko Kimura: Sure, how can I be of help?
Lisa Yamanaka: I am trying to write a paper on AIDS treatment in Japan, but I need more information. Can you (   )?
Yoko Kimura: OK, but I can't today. I have plans to meet friends for a study session.
Lisa Yamanaka: Another midterm exam?
Yoko Kimura: Yeah. This time I have to study for a (   ) test.
Lisa Yamanaka: Good luck! So how about tomorrow afternoon? Are you free then?
Yoko Kimura: (   ). We could have lunch together and then go to the library.
Lisa Yamanaka: Great. (   ) waiting for you. Study hard!
Yoko Kimura: I will! Bye.

Now work with your partner and try to say the above dialog (in natural English), but use your own words. For example, instead of "pharmacokinetics," you could say, "biology."

Naturally Spoken English Notes:

afternoon ＝ afdernoon   together ＝ tagether   waiting ＝ waiding

---

COLUMN

食品の分類

最近の国民の健康に対する高い関心からか，健康食品と称するさまざまな商品が出回っている．それではそもそも食品とはいかに分類されるものなのか．食品は，国が健康の保持増進効果を確認した"**保健機能食品**"とそれ以外の"**一般食品**"に分けられる．"保健機能食品"には"**特定保健用食品**"と"**栄養機能食品**"があり，前者，いわゆる特保は"からだの生理学的機能などに影響を与える保健機能成分を含む食品で特定の保健用途に資する旨を表示するもの"で，たとえば○○が含まれるのでおなかの調子を整えます，といった表示がある．一方後者は，"栄養素の補給のために利用される食品で栄養素の機能を表示するもの"で，カルシウムは骨や歯の形成に必要な栄養素です，といった表示がある．これらの表示は一般食品には認められておらず，健康食品といわれる食品が"保健機能食品"であるかどうかは，商品の表示を見れば一目瞭然ということになる．ただし一般食品であっても，基準にしたがった栄養成分の表示や栄養成分が含まれていることを<u>強調した</u>表示は可能となっている．

（平田收正）

Chapter 9

Bacteria, Viruses, and Antibiotics

Objectives

After studying this chapter, you should be able to:

- Read simple written sentences and identify the main idea in a timely fashion. [SBO 1]
- Explain the content of simple written passages in Japanese or English. [SBO 2]
- Explain what bacteria, viruses, and antibiotics are in English or Japanese. [SBO 3]
- Correctly explain English written for the sciences and related to clinical practice in Japanese or English. [SBO 4]
- Utilize one of the basic grammatical rules, postmodification, for reading and writing. [SBOs 2, 4, 5]
- Rewrite short Japanese sentences about Japanese culture and campus life into English without grammatical errors. [SBO 5]
- Outline the results of a simple chart in English. [SBO 8]
- Explain the content of English, including technical terms, related to pharmacy in Japanese or English. [SBO 3]
- Write a simple paragraph related to the sciences or clinical practice in English. [SBO 9]
- Tell the difference between sounds in spoken English. [SBO 10]
- Correctly pronounce the names of illnesses, parts of the body, and drugs. [SBO 13]

対応 SBO
SBOs 1,2,3,4

9・1 Reading

> ペニシリン（最初の抗生物質）の発見以来，細菌による感染症から多くの人々の命が救われてきた．しかし，近年，抗生物質が効かないという状況が生まれてきた．細菌の反逆だ．それは抗生物質の用い方にも問題があるようだ．今，科学的な視点から易しく細菌の反逆が解き明かされる．一緒に見ていこう．

CD
Track 17

What Are Bacteria and Viruses?

Bacteria are single-celled organisms usually found all over the inside and outside of our bodies, except in the blood and spinal fluid. Many

spinal fluid　（脊）髄液

bacteria are not harmful. In fact, some are actually beneficial. However, disease-causing bacteria trigger illnesses. Viruses are even smaller than bacteria. A virus cannot survive outside the body's cells. It causes illnesses by invading healthy cells and reproducing.

What Is an Antibiotic?

Antibiotics, also known as antimicrobial drugs, are drugs that fight infections caused by bacteria. Alexander Fleming discovered the first antibiotic, penicillin, in 1927. After the first use of antibiotics in the 1940s, they transformed medical care and dramatically reduced illness and death from infectious diseases.

The term "antibiotic" originally referred to a natural compound produced by a fungus or another microorganism that kills bacteria which cause disease in humans or animals. Some antibiotics may be synthetic compounds (not produced by microorganisms) that can also kill or inhibit the growth of microbes. Technically, the term "antimicrobial agent" refers to both natural and synthetic compounds. Although antibiotics have many beneficial effects, their use has contributed to the problem of antibiotic resistance.

What Is Antibiotic Resistance and Why Are Bacteria Becoming Resistant to Antibiotics?

Antibiotic resistance is the ability of bacteria or other microbes to resist the effects of an antibiotic. Antibiotic resistance occurs when bacteria change in some way that reduces or eliminates the effectiveness of drugs, chemicals, or other agents designed to cure or prevent infections. The bacteria survive and continue to multiply causing more harm. Bacteria can do this through several mechanisms. Some bacteria develop the ability to neutralize the antibiotic before it can do harm, others can rapidly pump the antibiotic out, and still others can change the antibiotic attack site so it cannot affect the function of the bacteria.

Antibiotics kill or inhibit the growth of susceptible bacteria. Sometimes one of the bacteria survives because it has the ability to neutralize or escape the effect of the antibiotic; that one bacterium can then multiply and replace all the bacteria that were killed off. Exposure to antibiotics therefore provides selective pressure, which makes the surviving bacteria more likely to be resistant. In addition, bacteria that were at one time susceptible to an antibiotic can acquire resistance through mutation of their genetic material or by acquiring pieces of DNA that code for the resistance properties from other bacteria. The DNA that codes for resistance can be grouped in a single easily transferable package. This means that bacteria can become resistant to many antimicrobial agents because of the transfer of one piece of DNA.

How Can I Prevent Antibiotic-resistant Infections?

Only use antibiotics when they are likely to be beneficial. Some useful tips to remember are:

1. Do not take an antibiotic for a viral infection like a cold or the flu.
2. Do not save some of your antibiotic for the next time you get sick. Discard any leftover medication once you have completed your prescribed course of treatment.
3. Take an antibiotic exactly as the healthcare provider tells you. Do not skip doses. Complete the prescribed course of treatment even if you are feeling better. If treatment stops too soon, some bacteria may survive and re-infect.
4. Do not take antibiotics prescribed for someone else. The antibiotic may not be appropriate for your illness. Taking the wrong medicine may delay correct treatment and allow bacteria to multiply.

5. If your healthcare provider determines that you do not have a bacterial infection, ask about ways to help relieve your symptoms. Do not pressure your provider to prescribe an antibiotic.

出典：© Centers for Disease Control and Prevention, http://www.cdc.gov/getsmart/antibiotic-use/anitbiotic-resistance-faqs.html（2010年12月1日現在）.

9・2 Reading Comprehension

Do the following statements agree with the information given in the passage? Write T in the bracket if the statement agrees with the information. Write F if it does not.

対応 SBO
SBOs 1,2,4,9

1. As they can cause infectious diseases, bacteria and viruses do more harm than good. (　　)
2. Antibiotic resistance occurs through the same mechanism to change the bacterial property. (　　)
3. If one of the bacteria survives antibiotic agents, it can acquire resistance to them. (　　)
4. Selective pressure prevents bacteria from continuing to multiply. (　　)
5. Genetic mutation can be involved when bacteria susceptible to an antibiotic become resistant to it. (　　)

9・3 Grammatical Rule：後置修飾（Postmodification）

対応 SBO
SBOs 2,4,5

形容詞には限定用法と叙述用法がある．限定用法とは，a *beautiful* sky のように名詞の前に置かれ修飾する用法のことであり，叙述用法とは，The sky is *beautiful* のように補語になるものをいう．

限定用法は，形容詞が名詞の前に置かれる場合と後ろに置かれる場合がある．後者を後置修飾という．自然科学の文章を読むためには後置修飾を正しく理解することが肝要である．

そこで，日本語と英語の語順を考えてみよう．

・私はそのケーキを食べたネズミを殺した猫と仲良しの犬を飼っている．
・I keep the dog that is getting along well with the cat that killed the mouse that ate the cake.

お気づきのとおり，日本語は前置修飾の言語であるのに対し，英語は後置修飾の言語である．後ろから訳さなくても意味が自然にとれるようになるまで，根気よく英語に慣れ親しむことが必要である．

では，本文中の次の英文を考えてみよう．後置修飾がいくつ使われているだろうか．

> The term "antibiotic" originally referred to a natural compound produced by a fungus or another microorganism that kills bacteria which cause disease in humans or animals.

54　9. Bacteria, Viruses, and Antibiotics

対応 SBO
SBOs 5,8

9・4　Writing

円グラフ（Pie Chart）の読み方を学ぼう．

例：(1) Ten percent of the international students are from Indonesia.
(2) International students from a few countries are enrolled at ABC University.

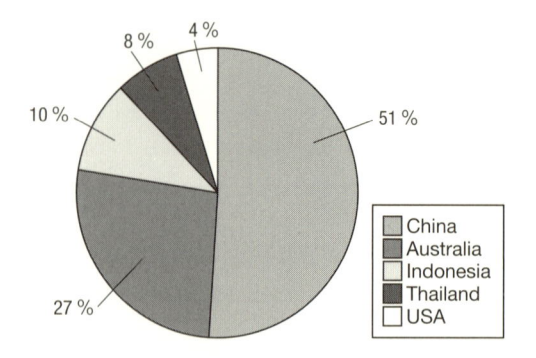

51 %
27 %
10 %
8 %
4 %

China
Australia
Indonesia
Thailand
USA

Number of International Students at ABC University in 2010

1. この円グラフから言えることを二つあげなさい．

   _____
   _____

2. あなたが学食の責任者だとすると，この表からどのような配慮をするか，書きなさい．

   If I were the manager of the school cafeteria, I ～

   _____
   _____

対応 SBO
SBOs 3,13

9・5　Medical Vocabulary

Write the name of each numbered part on the corresponding line.

(1) 瞼（まぶた）_____　(2) 涙腺 _____

(3) 瞳孔 _____　(4) 角膜 _____

(5) 網膜 _____

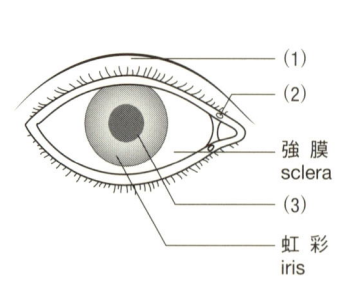

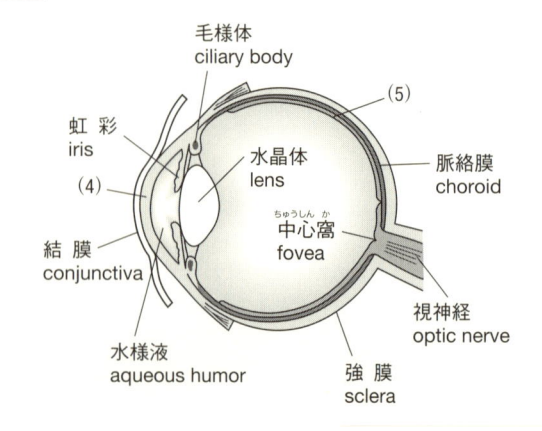

毛様体 ciliary body
虹彩 iris
水晶体 lens
中心窩（ちゅうしん か） fovea
結膜 conjunctiva
水様液 aqueous humor
脈絡膜 choroid
視神経 optic nerve
強膜 sclera

(1)
(2)
強膜 sclera
(3)
虹彩 iris

(4)
(5)

9・6 Listening/Speaking

▶ **Dictation**   Listen to the following conversation and fill in the blanks.

In front of the Professor's Office

Prof. Nagai：　　Lisa, (　　　　　　　　　　)! How have you been?
Lisa Yamanaka：　I'm OK. What's new with you, Prof. Nagai?
Prof. Nagai：　　(　　　　　　). I am too busy with meetings and committee work.
Lisa Yamanaka：　(　　　　　　　　　　　　　　) back in America.
Prof. Nagai：　　I am sure there isn't much difference. Anyway, where's Bruce?
Lisa Yamanaka：　I think he went to Akihabara with a student. Why?
Prof. Nagai：　　Well, (　　　　　　　　　) every Saturday morning and I would like you to pick an article and share it with the others.
Lisa Yamanaka：　OK, but today is Thursday.
Prof. Nagai：　　Well, (　　　　　　　　　　　) in the library yesterday?
Lisa Yamanaka：　As a matter of fact, I did. I have the perfect one in mind!

Now work with your partner and try to say the above dialog (in natural English).

Naturally Spoken English Notes：

　　article = ardicle　　today = taday

COLUMN

抗生物質とは

　1928年，A. Fleming はブドウ球菌を培養していて，培地に増殖した青カビの周りのブドウ球菌が溶けていることに気づき，ペニシリンを発見した．このペニシリンは，肺炎や化膿性疾患などで苦しんでいる多くの患者を救った．さらに，S. A. Waksman は土の中の微生物がつくるストレプトマイシンを発見して，多くの結核患者が救われた．Waksman は1941年に，"微生物によってつくられる化学物質で，低い濃度で他の微生物の発育を抑制したり，殺滅したりするもの" を**抗生物質** (antibiotics) と名づけようと提唱した．その後，多くの抗生物質が発見され，赤痢などの腸内感染症も治療できるようになった．また，悪性腫瘍（癌細胞）を死滅させる抗生物質なども発見されている．当初，抗生物質の発見により，人類は感染症の恐怖から解放されたといわれた．しかし，すぐに耐性菌の問題が起こってきた．その抗生物質に対して，微生物が変異を起こし，薬が効かなくなってしまったのである．そこで新たな抗生物質の探索や，化学合成した抗菌薬の開発研究が進められている．人類と細菌の戦いはいまだに続いているのである．

（笹津備規）

Chapter 10

Living with Parkinson's Disease

Objectives

After studying this chapter, you should be able to:

- Read simple written sentences and identify the main idea in a timely fashion. [SBO 1]
- Explain the content of simple written passages in Japanese or English. [SBO 2]
- Explain what is Parkinson's disease and how the drug for it works in English or Japanese. [SBO 3]
- Correctly explain English written for the sciences and related to clinical practice in Japanese or English. [SBO 4]
- Utilize one of the basic grammatical rules, participial construction, for reading and writing. [SBOs 2, 4, 5]
- Rewrite short Japanese sentences about Japanese culture and campus life into English without grammatical errors. [SBO 5]
- Write a simple paragraph related to the sciences or clinical practice in English. [SBO 9]
- Tell the difference between sounds in spoken English. [SBO 10]
- Summarize the understood content of an English conversation. [SBO 11]
- Correctly pronounce the names of illnesses, parts of the body, and drugs. [SBO 13]

対応 SBO
SBOs 1,2,3,4

CD
Track 19

* カナダ出身の有名な俳優，映画 "Back to the Future" で主演した．パーキンソン病の研究のため基金を設立．

siege
包囲攻撃，執拗な努力

embark 乗り出す

10・1 Reading

> パーキンソン病は中枢神経系の慢性的疾患である．原因は脳内の神経伝達物質の平衡失調であるとされている．米国では毎年 5 万人がパーキンソン病と診断され，現在 50 万人の患者がいる．研究によるとパーキンソン病患者は症状が現れる前にドーパミンを産生する細胞の 60〜80％を失っていることがわかっている．しかし，なぜどのようにしてそれらの細胞が死滅するのかはわかっていない．パーキンソン病の根本的病態の解明が期待されている．

Diagnosed with Parkinson's disease in 1998, actor Michael J. Fox* perhaps best captured the dramatic impact it can have when he said, "Parkinson's forced me to make a fundamental life decision: adopt a siege mentality—or embark upon a life journey."

Fox since has become one of the nation's foremost advocates for finding a cure for the disease, which was first described in 1817 by English physician James Parkinson as "the shaking palsy." In the early 1960s, researchers identified a fundamental brain defect that is the hallmark of PD: the loss of brain cells, or neurons, in an area known as the substantia nigra that produce dopamine, a chemical that helps direct smooth, purposeful muscle activity.

Subtle Onset of Classic Symptoms

Parkinson's disease produces a wide range of problems that appear and progress at different rates and to varying degrees from individual to individual. Early symptoms are often subtle and may include mild shaking of the limbs (tremor), slowness of movement or stiffness.

As the disease advances, four classic clinical signs typically appear:

- Tremor—rhythmic, back-and-forth trembling of the hands, arms, legs, jaw or face
- Rigidity—stiffness of the limbs and/or trunk
- Bradykinesia—the slowing down and loss of spontaneous and automatic movement, particularly frustrating because it may be unpredictable, and what once was routine, like washing or dressing, may take significantly longer
- Instability—impaired balance and stooped posture

Difficult to Diagnose

Typically a disease of late middle age, Parkinson's usually affects people over the age of 50, with 60 being the average age of onset. However, research over the last several years has demonstrated that as many as 10 percent of Parkinson's patients may experience onset before 40, like Michael J. Fox when he was diagnosed.

Even for experienced neurologists, accurately diagnosing Parkinson's in its early stages can be difficult in some cases. No blood or laboratory tests are available, so physicians may have to observe patients for some time until it is apparent that clinical signs and symptoms are consistent with a diagnosis of PD.

Effective Drug Relief

The primary therapy for PD is replacement of dopamine via levodopa (also called L-dopa, from the full name L-3,4-dihydroxyphenylalanine), a simple chemical found in plants and animals with which neurons can make dopamine to replenish the brain's dwindling supply; dopamine agonists, which mimic the role of dopamine in the brain; or a combination of both.

Introduced in the 1960s, levodopa relieves many troublesome symptoms of PD, extending the time in which the majority of patients can lead relatively normal, productive lives. (Dopamine itself cannot be given because it doesn't cross the blood-brain barrier, the elaborate meshwork of fine blood vessels and cells that filters blood reaching the brain.)

Causes

Researchers don't know why or how the cells die, but they are beginning to find fascinating new clues.

Free radicals: One theory holds that free radicals—unstable and potentially damaging molecules generated by the body's normal chemical reactions—may contribute to nerve cell death, thereby leading to Parkinson's in a process called oxidation. Evidence that oxidative mechanisms may cause or contribute to the disease includes the findings that Parkinson's patients exhibit increased brain levels of iron and decreased levels of ferritin, a protein that stores, or binds, iron in the body.

Environmental toxins: Some scientists have suggested that Parkinson's may occur from exposure to an environmental risk factor such as a pesticide or a toxin.

Genetics: A relatively new theory explores the role of genetic factors, since 15 to 25 percent of Parkinson's sufferers have a close relative who has experienced parkinsonian symptoms (such as a tremor).

出 典: NIH Medlineplus the magazine, Summer 2006 Issue, 14〜18, http://www.nlm.nih.gov/medlineplus/magazine/issues/summer06/articles/summer06pg14-18.html.（2010 年 12 月 1 日現在）より許可を得て転載.

10・2 Reading Comprehension

▶ **Question**　Answer the following questions in English.

対応 SBO
SBOs 1,2,4,9

1. How was Michael J. Fox diagnosed in 1998?

   _____

2. What instances are described as early symptoms of Parkinson's disease?

   _____

3. Why is it difficult for physicians to accurately diagnose Parkinson's disease in its early stages?

   _____

4. What is the primary therapy for Parkinson's disease?

   _____

5. What are cited as the causes for Parkinson's disease?

   _____

10・3 Grammatical Rule: 分詞構文 (Participial Construction)

対応 SBO
SBOs 2,4,5

分詞構文を覚えているだろうか．形は現在分詞句か過去分詞句であり，働きは主文の全体を修飾し，"時, 条件, 理由, 結果, 譲歩, 様態など"を表す副詞的用法である．
　分詞構文は，以下のように用いられる．

(1) 主文の前に置かれる場合
　　現在分詞句, S＋V＋...
　　(Being, Having の省略) 過去分詞句, S＋V＋...
(2) 主文の後ろに置かれる場合(科学論文では結果を表す頻度が高いようである)
　　S＋V＋..., 現在分詞句
　　S＋V＋..., (being, having の省略) 過去分詞句

では，下記の本文中の分詞構文はどのような意味を表しているか考えてみよう．

> **Diagnosed with the disease in 1998**, actor Michael J. Fox perhaps best captured the dramatic impact it can have when he said, "Parkinson's forced me to make a fundamental life decision: adopt a siege mentality—or embark upon a life journey."

10. Living with Parkinson's Disease

対応 SBO
SBO 5

10・4 Writing

趣味や娯楽に関する表現を学ぼう．

Michael J. Fox は数々の映画やテレビ番組で人気を得た．自分の趣味や好みの映画などについて下の質問に答えなさい．補足説明を加えて詳しく書きなさい．

1. What kind of movies do you like?
   （例）I like romantic movies. In particular, I like the movies of Audrey Hepburn, such as *Roman Holiday* and *Moon River*.

   _____

   _____

2. Do you like reading comic books?
   （例）I loved Doraemon when I was small and have seen all of the movies.

   _____

   _____

3. What is your favorite spectator sport?
   （例）I like watching baseball games. I am a big fan of the local team, the Jaguars, and I sometimes go to the ballpark to cheer on the players.

   _____

   _____

   _____

対応 SBO
SBO 13

10・5 Medical Vocabulary

Write the name of each numbered part on the corresponding line.

（1）樹状突起　_____　　（2）細胞体　_____

（3）核　_____　　（4）ミエリン　_____

（5）軸　索　_____

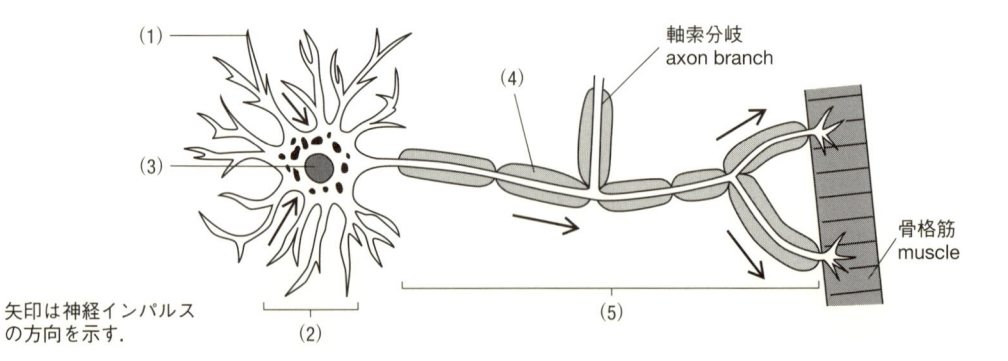

矢印は神経インパルスの方向を示す．
軸索分岐 axon branch
骨格筋 muscle

10・6 Listening/Speaking

▶ **Dictation**   Listen to the following conversation and fill in the blanks.

対応 SBO
SBOs 10,11,13
CD Track 20

In the Lab
Bruce Chen:　I'm back! Wow! (　　　　　　　　　　)! You have to go!
Lisa Yamanaka:　Well, (　　　　　　　　　　　　), you have to
　　　　　　　　take me next time. OK?
Bruce Chen:　(　　　　　　　　　　　　　　　)! What's wrong, you look
　　　　　　　　a <u>little</u> nervous.
Lisa Yamanaka:　Prof. Nagai stopped by yesterday and said we need to participate in
　　　　　　　　their journal club.
Bruce Chen:　They do journal club here, too? I didn't know that. When is it?
Lisa Yamanaka:　Tomorrow.
Bruce Chen:　Tomorrow!? Actually, I can present (
　　　　　　　　　　　　　). It's about drugs that help (
　　　　　　　　　　　　　).
Lisa Yamanaka:　You are so lucky! I was in the library all day yesterday looking.
Bruce Chen:　Well, I guess I am lucky. Anyway, (　　　　　　　　　　)?
Lisa Yamanaka:　Sure. Let's have a look.

Now work with your partner and try to say the above dialog (in natural English), but use your own words. For example, instead of "clinical pharmacology," and "suppress transplant rejection," you could say, "cell biology" and "cure acne."

Naturally Spoken English Notes:
　little = liddle

COLUMN

生命倫理 (Bioethics)

　すべての生命はやがて死を迎えるが，死の判定は必ずしも容易ではない．通常は心拍停止，呼吸停止，瞳孔散大の3所見を確認して死（心臓死）と判定される．医療技術が進んで，脳が完全に死んでいるが人工呼吸器により心臓や肺は動いている状態も起こりうるようになり，このような状態も"脳死"として人の死と判定されるようになり，多くの国民が死を考える機会となった．人の死をめぐっては，本人はもちろん，周りの家族や医療者にとっても最も大きな出来事であるため，さまざまな解決が難しい倫理的な問題を生じる．回復の見込みのない終末期や植物状態の患者に人工呼吸器，人工栄養などを用いて，生命を維持する延命治療の問題，こうした治療を拒否して人間としての尊厳を保って死を迎えようとする尊厳死や安楽死の問題．個々の患者の自己決定権と生命（生活）の質（QOL）を尊重して，生と死に真剣に向かい合い，患者中心の医療を支援することが医療にかかわるものの使命である．
　　　　　　　　　　　　　　　　　　（木内祐二）

Chapter 11
The Science of Drug Abuse & Addiction

Objectives

After studying this chapter, you should be able to:

- Explain what drug abuse and addiction is in English or Japanese. [SBO 2]
- Explain the content of English, including technical terms, related to pharmacy in Japanese or English. [SBO 3]
- Correctly explain English written for the sciences and related to clinical practice in Japanese or English. [SBO 4]
- Utilize one of the basic grammatical rules, concession, for reading and writing. [SBOs 2, 4, 5]
- Rewrite short Japanese sentences into English without grammatical errors. [SBO 5]
- Write a simple paragraph related to the sciences or clinical practice in English. [SBO 9]
- Tell the difference between sounds in spoken English. [SBO 10]
- Summarize the understood content of an English conversation between two pharmacy students. [SBO 11]
- Correctly pronounce the names of illnesses, parts of the body, and drugs. [SBO 13]

対応 SBO
SBOs 2,3

11・1 Reading

薬物乱用や薬物中毒は全世界的に広がる深刻な社会問題である．その害悪は計り知れないにもかかわらず，乱用は増大している．わが国では，平成5年度（1993年）より"6・26国際麻薬乱用撲滅デー"を広く普及し，薬物乱用防止"ダメ．ゼッタイ．"普及運動が実施されている．薬物乱用や薬物中毒にいたる仕組みは，脳の報酬系や神経伝達物質が関係する複雑なものである．重大犯罪を起こしたり，使用を止めても精神障害が持続することがある．

Understanding Drug Abuse and Addiction

drug abuse
薬物乱用，麻薬の乱用

compulsive せずにいられない，病みつきの，強迫的な

Many people do not understand why individuals become addicted to drugs or how drugs change the brain to foster compulsive drug abuse. They mistakenly view drug abuse and addiction as strictly a social problem and may characterize those who take drugs as morally weak. One very common belief is that drug abusers should be able to just stop taking drugs if they are only willing to change their behavior. What people often underestimate is the complexity of drug addiction—that it is a disease that impacts the brain and because of that, stopping drug abuse is not simply a matter of willpower. Through scientific advances we now know much more about how exactly drugs work in the brain, and we also know that drug addiction can be successfully treated to help people stop abusing drugs and resume their productive lives.

What Happens to Your Brain When You Take Drugs?

Drugs are chemicals that tap into the brain's communication system and disrupt the way nerve cells normally send, receive, and process information. There are at least two ways that drugs are able to do this: (1) by imitating the brain's natural chemical messengers, and/or (2) by overstimulating the "reward circuit" of the brain.

Some drugs, such as marijuana and heroin, have a similar structure to chemical messengers, called neurotransmitters, which are naturally produced by the brain. Because of this similarity, these drugs are able to "fool" the brain's receptors and activate nerve cells to send abnormal messages.

Other drugs, such as cocaine or methamphetamine, can cause the nerve cells to release abnormally large amounts of natural neurotransmitters, or prevent the normal recycling of these brain chemicals, which is needed to shut off the signal between neurons. This disruption produces a greatly amplified message that ultimately disrupts normal communication patterns.

Nearly all drugs, directly or indirectly, target the brain's reward system by flooding the circuit with dopamine. Dopamine is a neurotransmitter present in regions of the brain that control movement, emotion, motivation, and feelings of pleasure. The overstimulation of this system, which normally responds to natural behaviors that are linked to survival (eating, spending time with loved ones, etc.), produces euphoric effects in response to the drugs. This reaction sets in motion a pattern that "teaches" people to repeat the behavior of abusing drugs.

As a person continues to abuse drugs, the brain adapts to the overwhelming surges in dopamine by producing less dopamine or by reducing the number of dopamine receptors in the reward circuit. As a result, dopamine's impact on the reward circuit is lessened, reducing the abuser's ability to enjoy the drugs and the things that previously brought pleasure. This decrease compels those addicted to drugs to keep abusing drugs in order to attempt to bring their dopamine function back to normal. And, they may now require larger amounts of the drug than they first did to achieve the dopamine high—an effect known as *tolerance*.

Long-term abuse causes changes in other brain chemical systems and circuits as well. Glutamate is a neurotransmitter that influences the reward circuit and the ability to learn. When the optimal concentration of glutamate is altered by drug abuse, the brain attempts to compensate, which can impair cognitive function. Drugs of abuse facilitate nonconscious (conditioned) learning, which leads the user to experience uncontrollable cravings when they see a place or person they associate with the drug experience, even when the drug itself is not available. Brain imaging studies of drug-addicted individuals show changes in areas of the brain that are critical to judgment, decisionmaking, learning and memory, and behavior control. Together, these changes can drive an abuser to seek out and take drugs compulsively despite adverse consequences—in other words, to become addicted to drugs.

出 典：©National Institute on Drug Abuse, http://www.nida.nih.gov/Infofacts/understand.html（2010年12月1日現在）.

11・2 Reading Comprehension

▶ **Question** Circle T (true) or F (false) for each statement.

対応 SBO
SBOs 2,3,4

1. Drug abusers are morally weak and stopping drug abuse is a matter of willpower. (T , F)
2. Drug addiction can be remedied and people who quit abusing drugs can recover their active lives. (T , F)
3. Normal communication patterns between neurons are disrupted by the overwhelming surges in natural neurotransmitters caused by drugs. (T , F)
4. Drug abuse for a long period leads to alteration of appropriate glutamine concentration in the brain's chemical systems. (T , F)
5. The areas of the brain deeply involved in judgment, decisionmaking, learning and memory have been found to be affected by drugs. (T , F)

11・3 Grammatical Rule：譲歩（Concession）

対応 SBO
SBOs 2,4,5

英文法の用語に"譲歩"という言葉がある．譲歩とは"～にもかかわらず"という表現のことである．譲歩を表す表現には以下のようなものがある．

(1) Though (Although) S+V..., S+V...

(2) Even if S+V..., S+V...

(3) Whether S+V+ ～or～, S+V...

(4) No matter how/wh- S+V..., S+V...

(5) 形容詞・副詞 ＋as S+V..., S+V...
    Child as he is, he knows more than the average adult のように，無冠詞で名詞 Child を文頭に出す表現は，文法で習うことがあっても，現代ではほとんど使われることがない古い表現である．

(6) その他，in spite of, despite など

下記の英文では (5) の表現が使われている．どのような意味か考えてみよう．

> **Staggering as these numbers are**, however, they do not fully describe the breadth of the deleterious public health—and safety—implications, ...

11・4 Writing

対応 SBO
SBOs 5,9

意見や考えを表明する．

自分の意見や考えは I think it is because～ あるいは In my opinion, ～ などの表現を使うとよい．最初に日本語で考えてもよい．そのあと，文の構造を考えて英語にしてみよう．

11. The Science of Drug Abuse & Addiction

1. 日本では最近，若者たちの間に薬物汚染が広がっているといわれている．その原因は何だと思いますか．前述の語句で始め，自分の考えを述べなさい．

例）<u>I think it is because of</u> the prevalence of drug sales on the Internet.

_____
_____
_____
_____

2. この問題を解決するためにはどうしたらよいか，考えを述べなさい．

例）<u>In my opinion</u>, it is important to teach small children what drug abuse can lead to.

_____
_____
_____
_____

対応 SBO
SBOs 3,13

11・5 Medical Vocabulary

Write the name of each numbered part on the corresponding line.

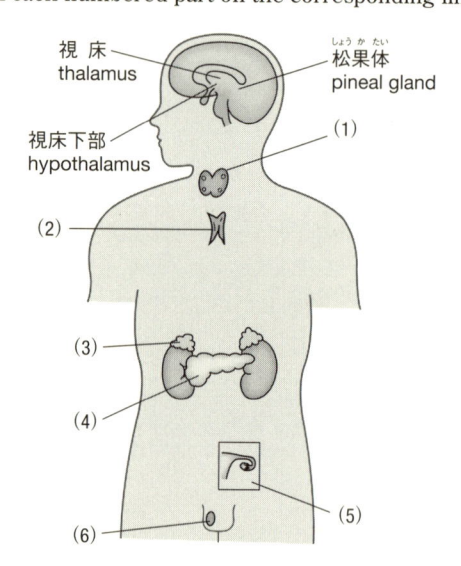

視床 thalamus
松果体 pineal gland
視床下部 hypothalamus

(1) 甲状腺 _____   (2) 胸腺 _____
(3) 副腎 _____   (4) 膵臓 _____
(5) 卵巣 _____   (6) 精巣 _____

11・6 Listening/Speaking

▶ **Dictation** Listen to the following conversation and fill in the blanks.

対応 SBO
SBOs 10,11
Track 21

In a Seminar Room

Yoko Kimura: Lisa, thanks for your presentation today. It was really interesting.
Lisa Yamanaka: You're welcome. (   ).
Yoko Kimura: But it was so professional. You were really prepared and had PowerPoint slides and everything.
Lisa Yamanaka: Actually, that's normal for us in pharmacy school in America. (   ).
Yoko Kimura: Really? It must be so difficult.
Lisa Yamanaka: (   ). But we must be prepared. The professors can ask some very tough questions.
Yoko Kimura: Do they tell you the questions in advance?
Lisa Yamanaka: No, (   ). Many times students can't <u>answer them</u>.
Yoko Kimura: Do they get angry with you?
Lisa Yamanaka: No, but we feel bad. Even after studying six, seven, or eight years, we see that (   ).

Now work with your partner and try to say the above dialog (in natural English).

Naturally Spoken English Notes:

a lot of = aladov   answer them = answer'em

COLUMN

ATPとミトコンドリア

　私たち哺乳類は真核生物（eukaryote）で，その細胞は遺伝情報であるDNAの格納庫である核など細胞内の分業工場である細胞内小器官（オルガネラ，organelle）をもっている．その一つであるミトコンドリア（mitochondrion［単］，mitochondria［複］）は生体エネルギー（bioenergy）の本体であるATP（アデノシン5'-三リン酸）をつくるエネルギーの発電所である．呼吸によって体内に取込んだ酸素を水に還元して，酸素がないときの20倍以上の効率でATPをつくる．

　実は，ミトコンドリアは20億年くらい前に真核生物の細胞に侵入し住み着いた細菌で，かつては自分自身の遺伝子でタンパク質を合成していた．しかし，細胞内に共生した今では，わずかに十数種のタンパク質しかつくらず，その機能を発揮するのに必要な残りのタンパク質は宿主から提供されたものを利用するようになった．

　私たちが1日に消費する約2000kcal程度のエネルギーに必要なATP量は300kg以上になるが，体内に存在しているATP量は数十グラム程度である．ミトコンドリアが休むことなく合成し続けたATPは，ADP（アデノシン5'-二リン酸）に分解されてエネルギーを放出し生命機能維持に用いられている．　　（寺田　弘）

Chapter 12

Allergies

Objectives

After studying this chapter, you should be able to:

- Read simple written sentences and identify the main idea in a timely fashion. [SBO 1]
- Explain the content of simple written passages in Japanese or English. [SBO 2]
- Explain what allergies are and how they affect our health in Japanese and English. [SBO 3]
- Correctly explain English written for the sciences and related to clinical practice in Japanese or English. [SBO 4]
- Utilize one of the basic grammatical rules, inanimate subject, for reading and writing. [SBOs 2, 4, 5]
- Rewrite short Japanese sentences about Japanese culture and campus life into English without grammatical errors. [SBO 5]
- Write a simple paragraph related to the sciences or clinical practice in English. [SBO 9]
- Explain the content of English, including technical terms, related to pharmacy in Japanese or English. [SBO 3]
- Tell the difference between sounds in spoken English. [SBO 10]
- Correctly pronounce the names of illnesses, parts of the body, and drugs. [SBO 13]

対応 SBO
SBOs 1,2,3,4

12・1 Reading

毎年，花粉症の季節になると憂鬱になる人がいる．アレルギーは数日で治るものではなく，患者のQOL（生活の質）に大きくかかわるものである．ここでは，アレルギーの症状と向き合う米国人の若者Gillianの手記と，アレルギーに関する基本的な情報を読んでみよう．

Allergies: Gillian's Story

　I was diagnosed with allergies when I was a little kid. Some people have mild allergies while others are unfortunate enough to have severe allergies that could even kill them. Although my allergies aren't that

severe, I am allergic to so many different things that they could really interfere with my life if I let them. Some of the things that affect me are pollen, animal dander, dust mites, and certain medications (like penicillin, which makes me swell up like a giant balloon!). I'm also
⁵ allergic to some foods.

I've been dealing with allergies for a long time now. I've been going to the allergist since I was 5 years old! I go every 2 weeks to get two shots, which really don't bother me at all. It's become a part of my life. I also take two different medications. As long as I get the shots and take my
¹⁰ medicines, I can pretty much carry on with my normal activities. It's all up to me whether I want to suffer or not!

Other than family, no one truly knows I have allergies, although I have to tell people it's allergies when my eyes start to tear up. I do get made fun of. Sometimes my buddies just tease in a friendly way, but kids I don't
¹⁵ know can bully me. I just ignore them. I often just tune them out by blasting my music. I also like to write in my journal or do yoga to work through any sad feelings.

You can't tell by looking at me that I have a health condition. I look like a normal kid, just like anyone else you would run into on the street. I
²⁰ don't mind telling people about my allergies — after all, it's normal to have them.

What Are Allergies?

Allergies are abnormal immune system reactions to things that are typically harmless to most people. When you're allergic to something,
²⁵ your immune system mistakenly believes that this substance is harmful to your body. (Substances that cause allergic reactions, such as certain foods, dust, plant pollen, or medicines, are known as **allergens**.)

In an attempt to protect the body, the immune system produces **IgE antibodies** to that allergen. Those antibodies then cause certain cells in

dust mites　ダニ

allergist
アレルギー専門医

tune out　＝ ignore

IgE　（＝Immuno-globulin E)　免疫グロブリンE

the body to release chemicals into the bloodstream, one of which is **histamine**.

The histamine then acts on the eyes, nose, throat, lungs, skin, or gastrointestinal tract and causes the symptoms of the allergic reaction. Future exposure to that same allergen will trigger this antibody response again. This means that every time you come into contact with that allergen, you'll have an allergic reaction.

Allergic reactions can be mild, like a runny nose, or they can be severe, like difficulty breathing. An asthma attack, for example, is often an allergic reaction to something that is breathed into the lungs by a person who is susceptible.

Some types of allergies produce multiple symptoms, and in rare cases, an allergic reaction can become very severe—this severe reaction is called **anaphylaxis**. Signs of anaphylaxis include difficulty breathing, difficulty swallowing, swelling of the lips, tongue, and throat or other parts of the body, and dizziness or loss of consciousness.

Anaphylaxis usually occurs minutes after exposure to a triggering substance, such as a peanut, but some reactions might be delayed by as long as 4 hours. Luckily, anaphylactic reactions don't occur often and can be treated successfully if proper medical procedures are followed.

出 典：©1995-2010 The Nemours Foundation, http://teenshealth.org/teen/diseases_conditions/allergies_immune/allergies.html#（2010年12月1日現在）より許可を得て転載．

12・2　Reading Comprehension

Do the following statements agree with the information given in the passage? Write **T** in the bracket if the statement agrees with the information. Write **F** in the bracket and rewrite the sentence so that it agrees with the information on the passage.

1. Gillian has been going to an allergist about every other week since she was five.　（　　）
2. Gillian's friends know that she is allergic to a few things.　（　　）
3. Substances that cause allergic reactions are called antibodies.　（　　）

4. An extreme case of anaphylaxis is dizziness or loss of consciousness. (　　)
5. Anaphylaxis may occur a few hours after a triggering substance enters the body, and it is possible that it may not cause any reactions. (　　)

▶ **Discussion Question**
What do you think of Gillian's Story?　Write a comment in Japanese or English.

_____

_____

_____

12・3　Grammatical Rule：無生物主語（Inanimate Subject）

対応 SBO
SBOs 2,4,5

この章の本文は二つの文体で書かれている．前半は，米国人の若者がアレルギーとどう向き合ったかを一人称の視点から情緒的に心情を告白している．後半は，アレルギーの機序について客観的に論じている．したがって，文の主語がすべて三人称である．換言すれば，前半が文学的文章で，後半が自然科学的文章であるといえよう．

自然科学の英文は，客観的に事実を描写する性質上，主語が三人称であることが多い．とりわけ，主語に"無生物主語"が用いられることがある．"文の主語に人間・生き物以外のもの，すなわち無生物を用いる"構文を無生物主語構文とよび，これは日本語にはない英語の特色をなす表現であるので，文意を解釈するときには十分気をつけなければならない．

では，下記の本文中の例文を見てみよう．どのような意味か考えてみよう．

Future exposure to that same allergen will trigger this antibody response again.
S　　　　　　　　　　　　　　　　V　　　　　　　　　O

幸い，この文の後に易しく言い換えた文が続いているので参考になる．
This means that *every time you come into contact with that allergen, you'll have an allergic reaction.*

12・4　Writing

対応 SBO
SBOs 5,9

Grammatical Rule を参考に，次の文を二通りの主語で書きなさい．

1. このお薬を飲むと，眠くなるかもしれません．

　This medicine may _____

　You may _____

2. 渋滞（traffic jam）に巻き込まれたため，バスは 2 時間遅れて駅に到着した．

_____

_____

12. Allergies

3. この実験により，私の仮説（hypothesis）が正しかったことが証明できるでしょう．

___

対応 SBO
SBOs 3,13

12・5　Medical Vocabulary

Write the name of each numbered part on the corresponding line.

(1) 咽頭　_____
(2) 喉頭　_____
(3) 気管　_____
(4) 気管支　_____
(5) 肺　_____

鼻 nose
胸膜 pleura

対応 SBO
SBO 10

CD Track 22

12・6　Listening/Speaking

▶ **Dictation**　Listen to the following conversation and fill in the blanks.

In the Professor's Office

Prof. Nagai: (　　　　　　　　　　　　　). Would you like to climb Mt. Fuji?
Lisa and Bruce: Yes!
Prof. Nagai: (　　　　　　　　　　　　), so I think you should be fine.
Bruce Chen: Maybe Lisa is, (　　　　　　　　　　　　).
Lisa Yamanaka: That's true. I have been walking a lot since I got here. But Bruce isn't exactly an athlete.
Prof. Nagai: (　　　　　　　　　). But you will need good hiking shoes. Do you have them?
Lisa Yamanaka: I thought we would be climbing Fuji-san, so I have mine.
Bruce Chen: Same with me. (　　　　　　　　　　　　)?
Prof. Nagai: Then it's <u>settled</u>. I will let you know the exact day of the trip tomorrow. (　　　　　　　　　　).
Lisa and Bruce: Bye.

Now work with your partner and try to say the above dialog (in natural English).

Naturally Spoken English Notes:
pretty ＝ predy 　　　 settled ＝ sedled

COLUMN

一般名タクロリムスとマクロリムス？

　タクロリムス（商品名：プログラフ）は，肝，腎，骨髄移植時の拒絶反応抑制に用いられる代表的な免疫抑制薬である．軟膏はアトピー性皮膚炎の治療にも用いられている．1985年に筑波山麓の土壌中から発見された放線菌の一種である *Streptomyces tsukubaensis* から単離され，かつての藤沢薬品工業（現アステラス製薬）により開発された．ヘルパーT細胞においてFK506結合タンパク質（FK506はタクロリムスの開発コード名で有機化学者にはこの名のほうが有名）と複合体を形成してカルシニューリンの活性化を阻害し，細胞内情報伝達系を抑制してインターロイキン-2などのサイトカインの産生を抑える．この医薬品の一般名は，最初，免疫抑制薬のステムであるリムスに大環状化合物から採ったマクロを冠してマクロリムスと提案されたが，マクロはあまりにも化学的であるからふさわしくないとの理由から，しゃれたことには筑波山のTをとってタクロリムスと命名された．

（富岡　清）

Chapter 13

E. coli

Objectives

After studying this chapter, you should be able to:

- Read simple written sentences and identify the main idea in a timely fashion. [SBO 1]
- Explain the content of simple written passages in Japanese or English. [SBO 2]
- Explain what *E. coli* is and how it works in our body in English or Japanese. [SBO 3]
- Correctly explain English written for the sciences and related to clinical practice in Japanese or English. [SBO 4]
- Utilize one of the basic grammatical rules, can of possibility, for reading and writing. [SBOs 2, 4, 5]
- Rewrite short Japanese sentences about experiments into English without grammatical errors. [SBO 5]
- Outline the methods and results of a simple science experiment in English. [SBO 8]
- Write a simple paragraph related to the sciences or clinical practice in English. [SBO 9]
- Tell the difference between sounds in spoken English. [SBO 10]
- Correctly pronounce the names of illnesses, parts of the body, and drugs. [SBO 13]

対応 SBO
SBOs 1,2,3,4

13・1 Reading

> 1996年夏，大阪市を中心に腸管出血性大腸菌 O157 による食中毒が発生し，患者は 9000 人を超え，児童 3 人が亡くなった．この大腸菌は強い感染力をもち，"ベロ毒素" とよばれる毒素を生み，強い毒性をもちうる．O157 の特徴，感染源，治療法，予防対策について理解しよう．

E. coli 大腸菌（ドイツの小児科医 Theodor Escherich の名から）

Outbreaks of foodborne disease caused by *E. coli* (*Escherichia coli*) bacteria have become a serious problem in this country. *E. coli* O157:H7, one type of the bacteria, has caused illness and major disease outbreaks in the United States. The Centers for Disease Control and Prevention estimates 73,000 cases of infection with *E. coli* O157:H7 and 61 deaths occur in this country every year.

Overview

Hundreds of *E. coli* strains are harmless, including those that thrive in the intestinal tracts of humans and other warm-blooded animals. These strains are part of the protective microbial community in the intestine and are essential for general health. Other strains, such as *E. coli* serotype O157:H7, cause serious poisoning in humans. Cattle are the main sources of *E. coli* O157:H7, but these bacteria are also in other domestic and wild mammals.

In 1982, scientists identified the first harmful foodborne strain of *E. coli* in the United States. O157:H7 refers to chemical compounds found on the bacterium's surface. In 2007, it accounted for about 7% of gut-related diseases reported to health agencies in the United States. In addition to *E. coli* O157:H7, there are other serotypes of *E. coli*, named enterohemorrhagic *E. coli*, that cause the same serious illnesses.

E. coli O157:H7 can produce one or more kinds of poisons that can severely damage the lining of the intestines and kidneys. These types of bacteria, called Shiga toxin-producing *E. coli* (STEC), often cause bloody diarrhea and can lead to kidney failure, especially in young children or in people with weakened immune systems. Most illness has been associated with contaminated food or water, contact with an infected person, or contact with animals that carry the bacteria.

Transmission

The U.S. Department of Agriculture, Food Safety and Inspection Service's recall site lists food products contaminated with harmful *E. coli*. The most common contaminated foods and liquids that have caused *E. coli* outbreaks include:

- Undercooked or raw hamburgers
- Salami
- Produce such as spinach, lettuce, sprouted seeds
- Unpasteurized milk, apple juice, and apple cider
- Contaminated well water or surface water frequented by animals

Symptoms

STEC can cause the following symptoms:

- Nausea
- Severe abdominal cramps
- Watery or very bloody diarrhea
- Fatigue

STEC can also cause low-grade fever or vomiting. Symptoms usually begin from 2 to 5 days after eating contaminated food or drinking contaminated liquids. Symptoms may last for 8 days and most people recover completely from the disease.

Complications

Hemolytic uremic syndrome, a serious complication of STEC, can lead to kidney failure and death. Children are particularly prone to this complication, and HUS is the most common cause of acute kidney failure in North America. Blood transfusions and kidney dialysis, performed in the intensive care unit of a hospital, is needed to treat this life-threatening condition. About 8 percent of people with HUS have other lifelong complications, such as high blood pressure, seizures, blindness, paralysis, and the effects of having part of their intestines removed.

Research

NIAID-supported scientists, in collaboration with Japanese colleagues, discovered that antibiotic therapy did not improve the outcomes of children with bloody diarrhea. Some antibiotics were even harmful, resulting in the release of more bacterial toxins and an increased risk of severe complications, including kidney damage and subsequent HUS.

Researchers have sequenced the genome of *E. coli* O157:H7 and compared it with the genome of the harmless *E. coli* K12. Seventy percent of the two genomes are identical, and the genome of *E. coli* O157:H7 is about 30 percent larger than K12. As researchers compare and contrast these and other strains of *E. coli*, their ability to answer key questions in evolution and disease processes will become easier.

sequence アミノ酸の配列を決定する

出 典：©National Institute of Allergy and Infectious Diseases, "*E. coli*", Bethesda, MD; U.S. Department of Health and Human Services, March 19, 2010, http://www3.niaid.nih.gov/topics/ecoli（2010年12月1日現在）より許可を得て転載.

13・2 Reading Comprehension

▶ **Question**　Answer the following questions in English.

対応 SBO
SBOs 1,2,4,9

1. What parts of the human body do harmless *E. coli* strains thrive in?

   _____

2. What part of the body can be damaged by the poisons of *E. coli* O157:H7?

   _____

3. When do symptoms of Shiga toxin-producing *E. coli* begin after eating contaminated food?

   _____

4. What conditions can hemolytic uremic syndrome lead to?

   _____

5. How are the genome of *E. coli* O157:H7 and that of *E. coli* K12 identical?

   _____

13・3 Grammatical Rule：可能性の Can（Can of Possibility）

対応 SBO
SBOs 2,4,5

助動詞 can は，(1) 能力・可能（〜できる），(2) 許可（〜してよい）を最初に学習する．しかし，自然科学の英語を読んでいると，この意味では不自然な場合がしばしばある．それが (3) 可能性（ときにはありうる）を表す can である．
本文中の次の例文を参照してみよう．

> *E. coli* O157:H7 *can* produce one or more kinds of poisons that *can* severely damage the lining of the intestines and kidneys.

イタリック体の can はどちらも "起こりうる可能性" を表している．この can は，自然科学の理論・経験から導き出される "一般的な可能性" をいうのであって，今現実にこれから起こる可能性を示唆するものではない．

では，医療従事者が次のように言った場合の患者の反応はどうだろうか．

(a) I hate to tell you, but your illness can be irreversible.
(b) I hate to tell you, but your illness may be irreversible.

どちらもショックではあるが，(a) にはわずかな望みを抱くが，(b) ではショックで絶望してしまうであろう．

対応 SBO
SBOs 5,8

13・4 Writing

科学実験の操作の説明 —— 命令形 (1)

何かの手順や方法を説明するには，命令形を用い簡潔に表記する必要がある．簡単な実験の手順の説明を英語にしてみよう．

1. 水をビーカーに入れて火にかけ，沸騰するまで加熱しなさい．

　　_____
　　_____

2. この固体を溶かすためには，三角フラスコ (Erlenmeyer flask) を使いなさい．

　　_____
　　_____

3. もし固まり (lump) がなかなか溶けなかったら，ガラス棒 (glass rod) でかき混ぜなさい．

　　_____
　　_____

4. 溶液 (solution) をそのまましばらく室温 (room temperature) で置いておき，結晶を注意して観察しなさい．

　　_____
　　_____

対応 SBO
SBO 13

13・5 Medical Vocabulary

Write the name of each numbered part on the corresponding line.

(1) 食　道　_____　　(2) 胃　　　_____

(3) 十二指腸　_____　　(4) 肝　臓　_____

(5) 膵　臓　_____　　(6) 直　腸　_____

総胆管
common bile duct

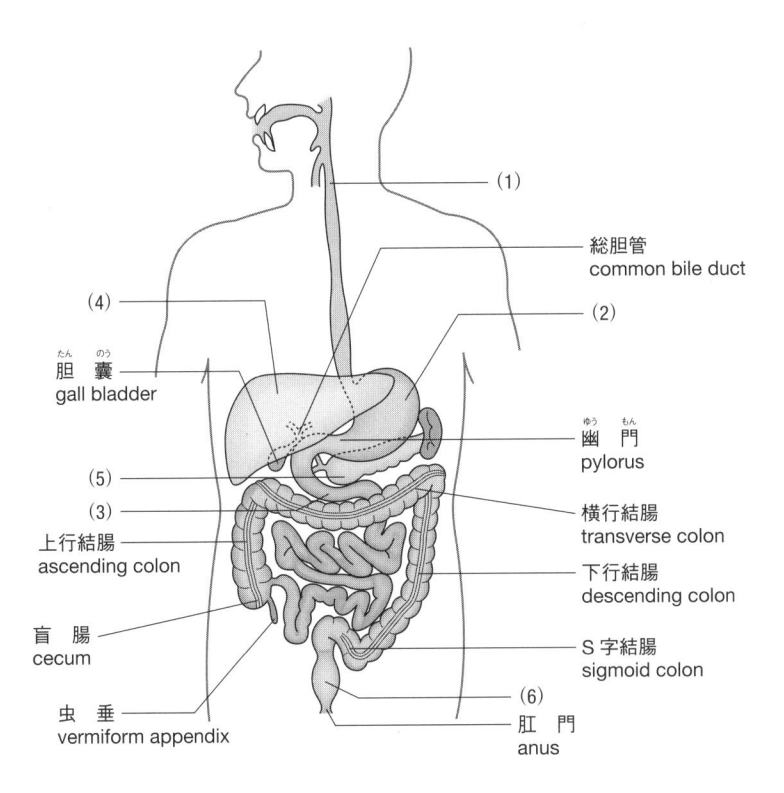

胆嚢
gall bladder

幽門
pylorus

横行結腸
transverse colon

下行結腸
descending colon

S字結腸
sigmoid colon

肛門
anus

上行結腸
ascending colon

盲腸
cecum

虫垂
vermiform appendix

13・6　Listening/Speaking

▶ **Dictation**　Listen to the following conversation and fill in the blanks.

対応 SBO
SBOs 10,13
CD Track 23

On Campus

Taro Yamada： Hey Bruce, what happened to your face?
Bruce Chen： (　　　　　　　　　　　　　　　). It really hurts!
Taro Yamada： Did you go to a drugstore for some cream?
Bruce Chen： (　　　　　　　　　　　　　　　). Everything's in Japanese.
Taro Yamada： If you want, I can go with you now. (　　　　　　　　　　　　).
Bruce Chen： Thank you so much! I think my face is on fire.
Taro Yamada： I think we can get you some cream with hydrocortisone in it. That should help.
Bruce Chen： And do you have Advil in Japan? (　　　　　　　　　　　　).
Taro Yamada： I'm sorry; I don't know what Advil is.
Bruce Chen： That's the brand name. (　　　　　　　　　　　　).
Taro Yamada： That we have. Let's go.

Now work with your partner and try to say the above dialog (in natural English).

Naturally Spoken English Notes:

did you ＝ didja　　I don't know ＝ I dunno

hydrocortisone ＝ hydracordizone　　ibuprofen ＝ aibuprofin

aspirin ＝ asprin

COLUMN

微生物と病気

　微生物が原因で起こる病気というと，思いつく病気は赤痢や肺炎などの"細菌感染"，インフルエンザやエイズなどの"ウイルス感染"，マラリアなどの"原虫・寄生虫感染"である．しかし，近年，これまで原因がわからなかった病気に微生物が関係していることがわかってきた．胃・十二指腸潰瘍は長い間，ストレスが原因であるといわれ，手術による患部の切除が行われていた．しかし，原因がヘリコバクター・ピロリという細菌であることがわかり，現在では抗菌薬による除菌と胃酸の分泌を止める薬の併用により治療されている．女性の子宮頸癌も，パピローマウイルスというウイルスの感染の結果，癌が発症することがわかり，予防のためのワクチン接種が行われている．血栓症に関しても，クラミジアという微生物が血管内に取りつき，血栓の核となっているのではないかという報告がある．このような例では，テトラサイクリンという抗菌薬を投与することにより，血栓症が治療される．このように，これまで原因がわからなかった病気の原因に，微生物が関係しているのではないかという研究が現在進められている．

（笹津備規）

Chapter 14

Report Calls for Clean Up of World's Dirtiest Dozen

Objectives

After studying this chapter, you should be able to:

- Read simple written sentences and identify the main idea in a timely fashion. [SBO 1]
- Explain what kind of pollution problems there are and how they are cleaned up in Japanese or English. [SBO 2]
- Explain the content of English, including technical terms, related to pharmacy in Japanese or English. [SBO 3]
- Correctly explain English written for the sciences and related to clinical practice in Japanese or English. [SBO 4]
- Utilize one of the basic grammatical rules, emphatic inversion, for reading and writing. [SBOs 2, 4, 5]
- Rewrite short Japanese sentences into English without grammatical errors. [SBO 5]
- Outline the methods and results of a simple science experiment in English. [SBO 8]
- Write a simple paragraph related to the sciences or clinical practice in English. [SBO 9]
- Tell the difference between sounds in spoken English. [SBO 10]
- Correctly pronounce the names of illnesses, parts of the body, and drugs. [SBO 13]

14・1 Reading

対応 SBO
SBOs 1,2,3,4

公害問題はかつて先進国の専売特許と思われていたが，現在では開発途上国へと広がり，国や地域を越えた地球規模での問題解決が求められている。この章では汚染浄化に努める非営利団体の取組みを報じる新聞の署名記事を読んでみよう。

By Burton Frierson

Reuters

NEW YORK — Twelve of the worst pollution problems in the

Reuters ロイター通信（英国の通信社．1851年設立）

developing world are being cleaned up, demonstrating that tens of thousands of others also could be improved, according to a report released last week.

The clean-up sites, ranging from Ukraine's Chernobyl nuclear disaster area to the polluted streets of Delhi, were in the fourth annual World's Worst Polluted Places Report issued by the New York-based Blacksmith Institute and Green Cross Switzerland.

In contrast to previous years' reports, which highlighted contaminated sites or specific pollution problems, the 2009 edition focused on clean-ups and solutions.

"Tens of thousands of polluted sites contaminate local populations — as many as 500 million people are poisoned each day in the developing world," the report said.

"Only a few of these problems have been fixed. But it's a start and worth recognizing."

The group's initial search for potential success stories yielded just 45 candidates. Making the final list were the only 12 cases that appeared to provide verifiable and credible evidence of success.

"Here we are talking about successes, but there's only 12 of them," Richard Fuller, president of Blacksmith Institute, told a teleconference of journalists.

"We've spent hundreds of billions of dollars in the West cleaning up our pollution problems here and at the same time we've shifted all our industry overseas and what we've done is ended up poisoning all these people in all these places overseas."

Blacksmith, an international not-for-profit organization, noted global progress in areas that were not geographically specific: removing lead from gasoline, which causes neurological damage, and efforts to eliminate through international treaty obsolete chemical weapons that maim and kill.

The report also listed 10 sites and what has been done to clean them up:

- Accra, Ghana: the broad commercialization of cooking stoves that reduce indoor air pollution, which causes respiratory illness in women and children;

- Candelaria, Chile: disposal of copper tailings and water treatment;

- Chernobyle-affected areas, Eastern Europe: medical, psychological and educational interventions to improve the lives of people in the zone of radiation contamination;

- Delhi: reduction of vehicle emissions that cause urban air pollution;

- Haina, Dominican Republic: removal of soil contaminated by the improper recycling of used car batteries, reducing lead levels in children's blood;

- Kalimantan, Indonesia: reduction of mercury poisoning from gold mining;

- Old Korogwe, Tanzania: removal of a stockpile of pesticides responsible for contaminating soil and a river;

- Rudnaya Pristan Region, Russia: removal of lead-contaminated soil in children's playgrounds;

- Shanghai: 12-year program to clean up sewage in an urban waterway that supplies drinking water to millions;

- West Bengal, India: reduction in arsenic poisoning through removal of naturally occurring arsenic in well water.

出 典: *The Daily Yomiuri*, November 6, 2009. トムソン・ロイター・マーケッツ株式会社より許可を得て転載.

Phasing Out Leaded Gasoline

Location	Global
Pollutant	Lead
Cause	The use of leaded gasoline to achieve higher octane ratings.
Health Impact	Lead poisoning causes central nervous system damage and impairs neurological development in children.
Output	Government agencies such as the U.S. EPA began to ban the use of leaded gasoline in the 70's; alternative fuels and other fossil fuel additives came into the market and became economically competitive at that time.
Outcome	As of February 2009, only eleven countries continue to use leaded gasoline and among these, only three used leaded gas exclusively.
Implications	Elevated blood lead levels among children dropped from 88 percent in the pre-phase out years to around 1 percent in the post-phase out years.
Remaining Challenges	Leaded gasoline is generally cheaper than its unleaded alternative. Developing nations with a lower quality of living often require government subsidies to implement a phase-out program.

出 典： © 2010 Blacksmith Institute, http://www.worstpolluted.org/projects_reports/display/66（2010 年 12 月 1 日現在）より許可を得て転載．

14·2 Reading Comprehension

▶ **Question**   Answer the following questions in English.

対応 SBO
SBOs 1,2,4,9

1. Who made the report about the world's worst polluted places?

   _____

2. What is the main difference between the 2009 edition and the previous years' reports?

   _____

3. Why are more people poisoned not in the West, but in the developing world?

   _____

4. What has been done to clean up the contamination of soil and a river in Tanzania?

   _____

5. Where and how was the project for removing lead from gasoline held?

   _____

14·3 Grammatical Rule：強調のための倒置（Emphatic Inversion）

対応 SBO
SBOs 2,4,5

英語は，先の5文型（p.41, §7·3参照）のような語順をとるのが常であるが，この語順の原則が破られることがある．倒置である．倒置には二つのタイプがある．

(1) 英語の慣用上行われる構文上の倒置   He loves her, and *so do I*.
(2) 語句を強調するための倒置   Not a word did she say to me.

では，本文中の例文を見てみよう．本来の語順に直すとどうなるか考えてみよう．

> *Making the final list* were the only 12 cases that appeared to provide verifiable and credible evidence of success.

14·4 Writing

対応 SBO
SBOs 5,8

科学実験の操作の説明 ── 命令形（2）

次の文章はニトロ化の実験の一部を説明したものである．カッコの中に適当な動詞を右の枠の中から選び書きいれなさい．必要に応じて大文字にしなさい．

(　　　) 9 cm³ of concentrated sulphuric acid into a boiling tube and (　　　) it below 10°C.

(　　　) a mixture of 3 cm³ of concentrated nitric acid with 3 cm³ of concentrated sulphuric acid in another boiling tube and (　　　) this mixture in the ice bath.

Use a dropping pipette to add the nitric acid and (　　　) the mixture to control the rate of addition.

When the addition is complete, (　　　) the reaction mixture over 40 g of crushed ice. (　　　) the product by suction filtration.

remove
cool
measure
add
stir
pour
collect

14. Report Calls for Clean Up of World's Dirtiest Dozen

対応 SBO
SBOs 3,13

14・5 Medical Vocabulary

Match the terms with their definitions and write the appropriate letter (a〜e) to the right of each term.

1. insulin　　　　　　　(　　)
2. GH (growth hormone)　(　　)
3. thyroid hormone　　　(　　)
4. epinephrine　　　　　(　　)
5. cortisol　　　　　　　(　　)

a. hormone that increases metabolic rate, influencing both physical and mental activities

b. hormone that is active in response to stress, increasing respiration, blood pressure, and heart rate

c. hormone that promotes growth of all body tissues

d. hormone that aids in metabolism of carbohydrates, proteins, and fats, and is active during stress

e. pancreatic hormone that regulates sugar metabolism

対応 SBO
SBO 10

CD
Track 24

14・6 Listening/Speaking

▶ **Dictation**　Listen to the following conversation and fill in the blanks.

In the Professor's Office

Lisa Yamanaka： Knock, knock. Prof. Nagai, are you free?
Prof. Nagai： Sure, Lisa, come on in.
Lisa Yamanaka： (　　　　　　　　　　　　　　　　). These are for you.
Prof. Nagai： Thank you so much, Lisa. (　　　　　　　　). By the way, where's Bruce? Is he OK?
Lisa Yamanaka： I think he went with one of the students to buy some medicine at a drugstore.
Prof. Nagai： I am glad to hear that. He got burned pretty bad. And (　　　　　　　　　　　　　　　)?
Lisa Yamanaka： It's <u>getting</u> there. Yoko has been helping me with the library resources. (　　　　　　　　　　　　).
Prof. Nagai： There weren't any in English? That's a shame.
Lisa Yamanaka： It's OK. (　　　　　　　　　　　　　　). Actually, I think it is helping her English.
Prof. Nagai： I am sure <u>it is</u>.

Now work with your partner and try to say the above dialog (in natural English).

Naturally Spoken English Notes：

getting ＝ gedding　　it is ＝ idiz

COLUMN

ファイトレメディエーション

　バイオレメディエーション，いわゆる生物的環境修復のなかで，植物の機能を利用するものを**ファイトレメディエーション**という．ファイト（phyto）は植物を表すギリシャ語に由来しており，植物がさまざまな物質を吸収・代謝する能力を利用して，土壌や水系から環境汚染物質を除去する方法である．対象物質は有害重金属，農薬や環境ホルモンといった有機化合物などがあり，おもに濃縮・分解，あるいは蒸散発により除去が行われる．本法では，物理・化学的処理に比べて低コストで低濃度・広範囲の汚染に対応可能なことや，実環境への適用が容易なことが利点であるが，処理速度が小さいことが最大の欠点であり，欧米に比べて，短期間での土地や水系の浄化が求められるわが国での普及は進んでいない．しかし，近年最終処分場面積が不足し，物理・化学的処理で生じる大量の汚染土壌や廃液の処分が難しくなっている．最近，遺伝子操作による浄化速度の上昇が可能になり，また環境ホルモンなどの浄化速度が大きい植物が発見されていることから，今後の本法の実用化が期待される．

〈平田收正〉

Chapter 15

A Drug's Life

Objectives

After studying this chapter, you should be able to:
- Explain what ADME is in English or Japanese.　　　　　　　　　[SBO 2]
- Explain the content of English, including technical terms, related to pharmacy in Japanese or English.　　　　　　　　　[SBO 3]
- Correctly explain English written for the sciences and related to clinical practice in Japanese or English.　　　　　　　　　[SBO 4]
- Utilize one of the basic grammatical rules, passive voice, for reading and writing.　　　　　　　　　[SBOs 2, 4, 5]
- Rewrite short Japanese sentences into English without grammatical errors.　　　　　　　　　[SBO 5]
- Outline the methods and results of a simple science experiment in English.　　　　　　　　　[SBO 8]
- Tell the difference between sounds in spoken English.　　[SBO 10]
- Ask and answer questions that come up in an English conversation.　　[SBO 12]
- Correctly pronounce the names of illnesses, parts of the body, and drugs. [SBO 13]

対応 SBO
SBOs 2,3

15・1　Reading

> "どうして薬を飲むと病気が治るのかと思って薬（薬学）に興味をもつようになった." という薬学生は少なくないだろう．実際，薬が人の体の中に入って，その役目を終えるまでの"薬の一生"はそんなに簡単ではないようだ．薬は体内で起こるさまざまな作用を事前に考慮してつくられるが，それ以上に人体は限りなく複雑で精巧につくられているようだ．ここでは"薬の一生"を一緒に見ていこう．

　Scientists have names for the four basic stages of a medicine's life in the body: absorption, distribution, metabolism, and excretion. The entire process is sometimes abbreviated ADME. The first stage is *absorption*. Medicines can enter the body in many different ways, and they are absorbed when they travel from the site of administration into the body's

site of administration
投与部位

circulation. A few of the most common ways to administer drugs are oral (swallowing an aspirin tablet), intramuscular (getting a flu shot in an arm muscle), subcutaneous (injecting insulin just under the skin), intravenous (receiving chemotherapy through a vein), or transdermal (wearing a skin patch). A drug faces its biggest hurdles during absorption. Medicines taken by mouth are shuttled via a special blood vessel leading from the digestive tract to the liver, where a large amount may be destroyed by metabolic enzymes in the so-called "first-pass effect." Other routes of drug administration bypass the liver, entering the bloodstream directly or via the skin or lungs.

Once a drug gets absorbed, the next stage is *distribution*. Most often, the bloodstream carries medicines throughout the body. During this step, side effects can occur when a drug has an effect in an organ other than the target organ. For a pain reliever, the target organ might be a sore muscle in the leg; irritation of the stomach could be a side effect. Many factors influence distribution, such as the presence of protein and fat molecules in the blood that can put drug molecules out of commission by grabbing onto them.

Drugs destined for the central nervous system (the brain and spinal cord) face an enormous hurdle: a nearly impenetrable barricade called the blood-brain barrier. This blockade is built from a tightly woven mesh of capillaries cemented together to protect the brain from potentially dangerous substances such as poisons or viruses. Yet pharmacologists have devised various ways to sneak some drugs past this barrier.

After a medicine has been distributed throughout the body and has done its job, the drug is broken down, or *metabolized*. The breaking down of a drug molecule usually involves two steps that take place mostly in the body's chemical processing plant, the liver. The liver is a site of continuous and frenzied, yet carefully controlled, activity. Everything that enters the bloodstream—whether swallowed, injected, inhaled, absorbed through the skin, or produced by the body itself—is carried to this largest internal organ. There, substances are chemically pummeled, twisted, cut apart, stuck together, and transformed.

The biotransformations that take place in the liver are performed by the body's busiest proteins, its enzymes. Every one of your cells has a variety of enzymes, drawn from a repertoire of hundreds of thousands. Each enzyme specializes in a particular job. Some break molecules apart, while others link small molecules into long chains. With drugs, the first step is usually to make the substance easier to get rid of in urine.

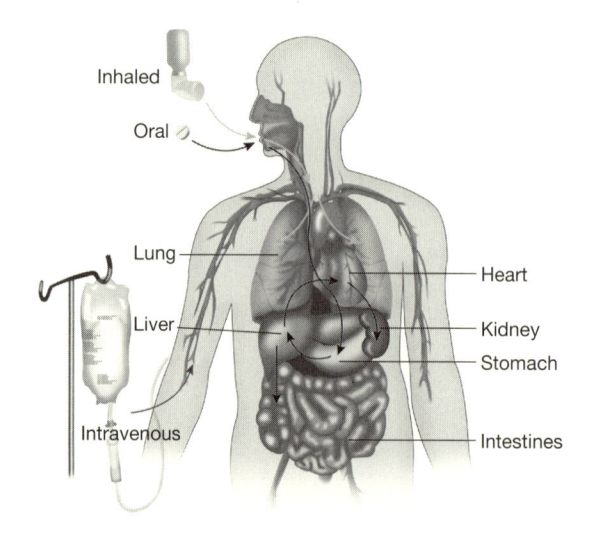

Figure 1　A Drug's Life in the Body　Medicines taken by mouth (oral) pass through the liver before they are absorbed into the bloodstream. Other forms of drug administration bypass the liver, entering the blood directly.

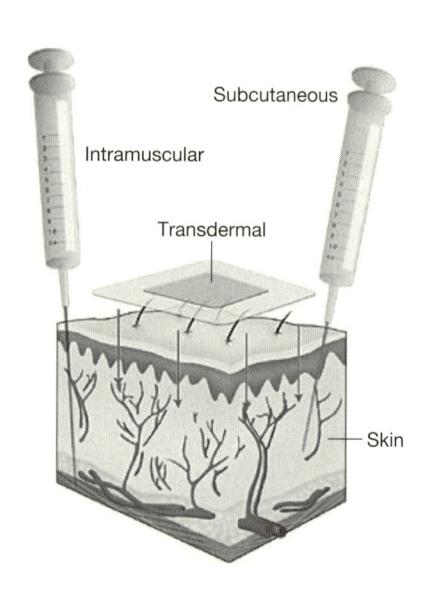

Figure 2　Drugs enter different layers of skin via intramuscular, subcutaneous, or transdermal delivery methods.

Many of the products of enzymatic breakdown, which are called metabolites, are less chemically active than the original molecule. For this reason, scientists refer to the liver as a "detoxifying" organ. Occasionally, however, drug metabolites can have chemical activities of their own—sometimes as powerful as those of the original drug. When prescribing certain drugs, doctors must take into account these added effects. Once liver enzymes are finished working on a medicine, the now-inactive drug undergoes the final stage of its time in the body, *excretion*, as it exits via the urine or feces.

feces　糞便

出 典：© National Institute of General Medical Sciences, *Medicines By Design*, p.5〜9, http://publications.nigms.nih.gov/medbydesign/medbydesign.pdf（2010 年 12 月 1 日現在）．

15・2　Reading Comprehension

▶ **Question**　Answer the following questions in English.

対応 SBO
SBOs 2,3,4

1. What does ADME stand for?

   _____

2. What happens in the "first-pass effect"?

   _____

3. What is the function of the blood-brain barrier?

   _____

4. Where does metabolism occur mostly?

   _____

5. What happens during the final stage of a drug's life in the body?

   _____

15・3　Grammatical Rule：受動態（Passive Voice）

対応 SBO
SBOs 2,4,5

英語には能動態（Active Voice）と受動態（Passive Voice）がある．

喜怒哀楽を表すのに受動態が用いられるのはゲルマン語の特徴であり，"死なれる"，"雨に降られる" などの "れる" は "迷惑の受身" といって自動詞が使われる．これは日本語の特徴の一つである．

一般的に能動態でも受動態でも同じ意味を表すことが可能である．

Watson and Crick discovered the DNA structure.　　　（能動態）
The DNA structure *was discovered* by Watson and Crick.　（受動態）

では，両者はどのように使い分ければよいのであろうか．換言すれば，受動態が望ましい理由はどのような場合であろうか．それは**文脈の流れ**による．下記の例文の主題が何であるかを考えれば容易に察しがつくであろう．

Do you know *who* discovered the DNA structure?　（主題は who）
Watson and Crick did.
*It was discovered by Watson and Crick.

15. A Drug's Life

では，本文中の次の例文では，なぜ受動態が使われているかを考えてみよう．

> Medicines can enter the body in many different ways, and **they are absorbed** when they travel from the site of administration into the body's circulation.

対応 SBO
SBOs 5, 8

15・4 Writing

科学実験の操作の説明 —— 受動態

実験器具に関する補足説明には受動態がしばしば用いられる．以下の語句に続けて文章をつくりなさい．

1. その器具を使用後すぐに洗っておくと，かなりの時間が省ける．
   Considerable time can be saved by

   _____

   _____

2. ビュレット（burette）を使うと少量の液体が測定できる．
   Small volumes of liquid

   _____

   _____

3. ガスバーナーは加熱やガラス細工（glasswork）に幅広く（extensively）使われる．
   A gas burner

   _____

   _____

対応 SBO
SBOs 3, 13

15・5 Medical Vocabulary

Match the terms with their meanings and write the appropriate letter (a～e) to the right of each term.

1. antineoplastic   (　　)   a. agent that suppresses seizures
2. corticosteroid   (　　)   b. agent that prevents blood clotting
3. sedative   (　　)   c. anti-inflammatory agent
4. anticonvulsant   (　　)   d. agent that destroys cancer cells
5. anticoagulant   (　　)   e. agent that induces relaxation

15・6 Listening/Speaking

▶ **Dictation** Listen to the following conversation and fill in the blanks.

対応 SBO
SBOs 10,12,13
CD Track 25

In the Lab

Bruce Chen： I'm back!

Lisa Yamanaka： (   ). Wow, you are really red!

Bruce Chen： Actually, Taro helped me find a good skin cream and I am taking some aspirin. (   ).

Lisa Yamanaka： Glad to hear it. We only have a few more days to go. (   ).

Bruce Chen： Yeah. Who knew Mt. Fuji could be so dangerous?

Lisa Yamanaka： Oh, by the way, Prof. Nagai was asking if there was somewhere we wanted to visit.

Bruce Chen： (   ). I went to a drugstore. You know, I wonder if we could visit a drug company?

Lisa Yamanaka： I was thinking the same thing. (   ).

Bruce Chen： And I am sure Prof. Nagai can <u>introduce</u> us to someone he knows.

Lisa Yamanaka： Let's go ask!

Now work with your partner and try to say the above dialog (in natural English).

Naturally Spoken English Notes：

　hospitals = hospidals　　pharmaceutical = pharmaceudical
　introduce = intraduce

Chapter 16

Anti-Cancer Drugs

Objectives

After studying this chapter, you should be able to:

- Explain what anti-cancer drugs are in English or Japanese. [SBO 2]
- Explain the content of English, including technical terms, related to pharmacy in Japanese or English. [SBO 3]
- Correctly explain English written for the sciences and related to clinical practice in Japanese or English. [SBO 4]
- Utilize one of the basic grammatical rules, case of the preposition "of," for reading and writing. [SBOs 2, 4, 5]
- Rewrite short Japanese sentences into English without grammatical errors. [SBO 5]
- Outline the methods and results of a simple science experiment in English. [SBO 8]
- Tell the difference between sounds in spoken English. [SBO 10]
- Summarize the understood content of an English conversation between four pharmacy students. [SBO 11]
- Ask and answer questions that come up in an English conversation. [SBO 12]
- Correctly pronounce the names of illnesses, parts of the body, and drugs. [SBO 13]

対応 SBO
SBOs 2,3

16・1 Reading

> 癌は急性心筋梗塞・脳卒中と並び三大疾病の一つである．わが国では1981年以来，癌が死亡原因の第1位となり，現在死因の約3割を占めている．世界中で，これまでさまざまな癌治療法が研究されてきており，効果的な化学療法剤の開発が進んでいる．最新の化学療法剤の種類と具体例，ならびに問題点について理解しよう．

chemotherapy
化学療法

Chemotherapy is a way to catch cancer cells that have spread. Unlike radiation, which treats only the part of the body exposed to the radiation, chemotherapy treats the entire body. As a result, any cells that may have escaped from where the cancer originated are treated. Most chemotherapeutic drugs kill cells by damaging their DNA or interfering with DNA synthesis. The hope is that all cancer cells will be killed, while leaving enough normal cells untouched to allow the body to keep functioning. Combining drugs that have different actions at the cellular level may help destroy a greater number of cancer cells. Combinations might also reduce the risk of the cancer developing resistance to one particular drug. What chemicals are used is generally based on the type of cancer and the patient's age, general health, and perceived ability to tolerate potential side effects. Some of the types of chemotherapy medications commonly used to treat cancer include:

Alkylating agents These medications interfere with the growth of cancer cells by blocking the replication of DNA.

Antimetabolites These drugs block the enzymes needed by cancer cells to live and grow.

Antitumor antibiotics These antibiotics—different from those used to treat bacterial infections—interfere with DNA, blocking certain enzymes and cell division and changing cell membranes.

Mitotic inhibitors These drugs inhibit cell division or hinder certain enzymes necessary in the cell reproduction process.

Nitrosoureas These medications impede the enzymes that help repair DNA.

Whenever possible, chemotherapy is specifically designed for the particular cancer. For example, in some cancers, a small portion of chromosome 9 is missing. Therefore, DNA metabolism differs in the cancerous cells compared with normal cells. Specific chemotherapy for the cancer can exploit this metabolic difference and destroy the cancerous cells.

One drug, taxol, extracted from the bark of the Pacific yew tree, was found to be particularly effective against advanced ovarian cancers, as well

microtubule　微小管（細胞内にみられる微小な管状構造物．近年抗癌剤の標的として注目されている．）
taxoid　タキソイド

leukemia　白血病
lymphoma　リンパ腫
testicular　こう丸の
combination chemotherapy　併用化学療法
Hodgkin disease　ホジキン病（悪性リンパ腫の一つ．頸部リンパ節や脾臓が腫れ，造血臓器が系統的に侵される病気．英国の病理学者T. Hodgkinが初めて報告．）

as breast, head, and neck tumors. Taxol interferes with microtubules needed for cell division. Now, chemists have synthesized a family of related drugs, called taxoids, which may be more powerful and have fewer side effects than taxol.

Certain types of cancer, such as leukemias, lymphomas, and testicular cancer, are now successfully treated by combination chemotherapy alone. The survival rate for children with childhood leukemia is 80%. Hodgkin disease, a lymphoma, once killed two out of three patients. Combination therapy, using four different drugs, can now wipe out the disease in a matter of months. Three out of four patients achieve a cure, even when the cancer is not diagnosed immediately. In other cancers—most notably, breast and colon cancer—chemotherapy can reduce the chance of recurrence after surgery has removed all detectable traces of the disease.

multidrug resistance　多剤耐性
plasma membrane carrier　細胞膜輸送体（細胞膜に存在する多種の膜タンパク質で，物質の輸送を担う．）

Chemotherapy sometimes fails because cancer cells become resistant to one or several chemotherapeutic drugs, a phenomenon called multidrug resistance. This occurs because a plasma membrane carrier pumps the drug (or drugs) out of the cancer cell before it can be harmed. Researchers are testing drugs known to poison the pump in an effort to restore the effectiveness of the drugs. Another possibility is to use combinations of drugs with different toxic activities, because cancer cells can't become resistant to many different types at once.

出典：Sylvia S. Mader, "*Human Biology*", 11th Ed. (International Student Edition), p.457〜459, The McGraw-Hill Companies, Inc. (2010) より許可を得て転載．

対応 SBO
SBOs 2,3,4

16・2　Reading Comprehension

▶ **Question**　Circle T (true) or F (false) for each statement.

1. A patient's overall health condition should be taken into account when choosing chemicals used in chemotherapy.　　　　　　　　　　　　　　(T , F)
2. A small percentage of child victims of leukemia cannot survive with the treatment of combination therapy.　　　　　　　　　　　　　　(T , F)

3. Enzymes that are crucial in cell reproduction can be hindered by mitotic inhibitors. (T , F)
4. Plasma membrane carriers are not involved in the development of resistance to chemotherapeutic drugs. (T , F)
5. Nitrosoureas help increase the enzymes which contribute to DNA repair. (T , F)

16・3 Grammatical Rule： 前置詞 of の格
(The Case of the Preposition "of")

対応 SBO
SBOs 2,4,5

前置詞 of を "〜の" と訳すことを覚え，それに終始するとうまく意味がとれないことがある．of の基本的な意味は，off と語源は同じで "分離" である．そして，位置，出所，起源の分離，全体から分離した部分，材料，所属などを表す．

自然科学の英語を読む際は，次のような of の用法に注意する必要がある．前置詞 of の左右に置かれた語句の意味関係をよく考えて，解釈することが重要である．

(1) 所有格　Aspirin is property *of* a German company.
　　　　　（＝A company owns the property.）

(2) 主　格　We all believe in the success *of* the team.
　　　　　（＝The team will succeed.）

(3) 目的格　We should respect her love *of* biology.
　　　　　（＝She loves biology.）

(4) 同　格　I admire her idea *of* loving patients.
　　　　　（＝her idea that she loves patients.）

では，次の本文中の例文を見てみよう．何格の of であろうか．

> Combinations might also reduce the risk ***of*** the cancer developing resistance to one particular drug.

16・4 Writing

対応 SBO
SBOs 5,8

実験結果の説明をしてみよう．

§12・3 (p.71) の無生物主語やこれまで学んだことを参考に，以下を英語にしなさい．

1. 操作の結果，リトマス試験紙 (litmus paper) が赤色に変わった．

_____

_____

2. その溶液を摂氏5℃まで冷やしたところ，澄んだ青色に変わった．

_____

_____

3. フラスコの中の残留物（residue）からは，この物質が純粋であるかどうかはわからなかった．

_____
_____

4. 硝酸（nitric acid）のOH^-イオンが脱離することによってNO_2^+イオンができた．

_____
_____

16・5 Medical Vocabulary

Match the terms with their definitions and write the appropriate letter（a〜e）to the right of each term.

1. erythrocyte   (　　)   a. a blood platelet
2. leukocyte   (　　)   b. a red blood cell
3. lymphocyte   (　　)   c. the liquid portion of the blood
4. thrombocyte   (　　)   d. a lymphatic cell
5. plasma   (　　)   e. a white blood cell

16・6 Listening/Speaking

▶ **Dictation**   Listen to the following conversation and fill in the blanks.

In the Lab
Bruce Chen:　　Well, Taro, (　　　　　　　　　　　　　　　　　).
Taro Yamada:　　You are welcome. It was nice to make a new friend.
Lisa Yamanaka:　And thank you, Yoko. (　　　　　　　　　　　　)!
Yoko Kimura:　　It was a pleasure! By the way, do you know how to get back to the airport tomorrow?
Bruce Chen:　　(　　　　　　　　　　　　　　　　), but do you have a better idea?
Taro Yamada:　　Yoko and I were talking and thought we would go with you to the airport. Tomorrow is Sunday and we have time.
Lisa Yamanaka:　That would be great! (　　　　　　　　　　). What time do you think we should leave here?
Yoko Kimura:　　I think (　　　　　　　　　　　), so we should leave at about noon. We need to go to Shinjuku and change trains.
Bruce Chen:　　I agree. I checked the schedule online and (　　　　　　　　　　　　　　　　).
Taro Yamada:　　OK. (　　　　　　　　　　　　　　). See you tomorrow.

Now work with your partner and try to say the above dialog (in natural English).

Naturally Spoken English Notes:
better = beder

COLUMN

悪魔の薬が，命の薬に

　1957年に旧西ドイツで開発された**サリドマイド**は，誤って多量服用しても死亡することのない安全な睡眠薬として汎用された．その当時，先天性胎児奇形である四肢の欠損が目立つ"あざらし肢症"が急増し，妊娠初期の"つわり"に悩む女性が服用したサリドマイドとの因果関係が疫学的調査から明らかになった．その後，サリドマイドは製造中止，1961年に市場から回収されることになったが，残念ながら，わが国で回収作業が終了したのはその2年後となり，多くの被害が出た．いったんは世の中から消え去ったサリドマイドであるが，近年，薬害をひき起こしたサリドマイドの特異な薬理作用（血管新生抑制，細胞増殖因子の産生抑制，細胞死の誘導など）を逆手にとって，既存薬が効果不十分な難病（ハンセン氏病，AIDS，多発性骨髄腫など）の治療薬としての利用が注目されている．わが国でも，"サリドマイド製剤安全管理手順"の遵守を条件に，多発性骨髄腫治療薬としてサリドマイドの使用が2008年に承認された．数奇な運命をたどった"悪魔の薬サリドマイド"は，私たちに多くの教訓を与え，今まさに，難病で苦しむ患者にとっては"命の薬"としてよみがえったことになる．

　　　　　　　　　　　　　　　　（入江徹美）

Chapter 17

Medicines for the Future

Objectives

After studying this chapter, you should be able to:

- Explain the content of simple written passages in Japanese or English. [SBO 2]
- Explain in English or Japanese how different it is to take today's medicines from medicines in the future. [SBO 3]
- Correctly explain English written for the sciences and related to clinical practice in Japanese or English. [SBO 4]
- Utilize one of the basic grammatical rules, parenthesis, for reading and writing. [SBOs 2, 4, 5]
- Rewrite short Japanese sentences about Japanese culture and campus life into English without grammatical errors. [SBO 5]
- Outline the methods and results of a simple science experiment in English. [SBO 8]
- Summarize the understood content of an English conversation. [SBO 11]
- Answer questions about a short explanation on pharmacy practice in English. [SBO 12]
- Correctly pronounce technical terms related to medication. [SBO 13]

対応 SBO
SBOs 2,3

17・1 Reading

> あなたは"2050年処方箋の旅"を想像できるだろうか．とは言っても，SF（空想科学小説）の世界ではない．人間という小宇宙に飛び出す薬を乗せた宇宙船の話だ．誰にでもおおむね効く薬から，ひとりひとりに的確に効く薬が生まれようとしている．そのカギを握るのはDNAだ．遺伝子科学は私たちに何をもたらしてくれるのだろうか．最前線をのぞいてみよう．

A Visit to the Doctor

May 17, 2050—You wake up feeling terrible, and you know it's time to see a doctor. In the office, the physician looks you over, listens to your symptoms, and prescribes a drug. But first, the doctor takes a look at your DNA.

symptom 症状，兆候
prescribe a drug
薬を処方する

That's right, your DNA. Researchers predict that the medicines of the future may not only look and work differently than those you take today, but tomorrow's medicines will be tailored to your genes. In 10 to 20 years, many scientists expect that genetics—the study of how genes influence actions, appearance, and health—will pervade medical treatment. Today, doctors usually give you an "average" dose of a medicine based on your body size and age. In contrast, future medicines may match the chemical needs of your body, as influenced by your genes. Knowing your unique genetic make-up could help your doctor prescribe the right medicine in the right amount, to boost its effectiveness and minimize possible side effects.

Along with these so-called pharmacogenetic approaches, many other research directions will help guide the prescribing of medicines. The science of pharmacology—understanding the basics of how our bodies react to medicines and how medicines affect our bodies—is already a vital part of 21st-century research.

21st-Century Science

While strategies such as chemical genetics can quicken the pace of drug discovery, other approaches may help expand the number of molecular targets from several hundred to several thousand. Many of these new avenues of research hinge on biology.

Relatively new brands of research that are stepping onto center stage in 21st-century science include genomics (the study of all of an organism's genetic material), proteomics (the study of all of an organism's proteins), and bioinformatics (using computers to sift through large amounts of biological data). The "omics" revolution in biomedicine stems from biology's gradual transition from a gathering, descriptive enterprise to a science that will someday be able to model and predict biology. If you

17. Medicines for the Future

think 25,000 genes is a lot (the number of genes in the human genome), realize that each gene can give rise to different variations of the same protein, each with a different molecular job. Scientists estimate that humans have hundreds of thousands of protein variants. Clearly, there's lots of work to be done, which will undoubtedly keep researchers busy for years to come.

A Chink in Cancer's Armor

Recently, researchers made an exciting step forward in the treatment of cancer. Years of basic research investigating circuits of cellular communication led scientists to tailor-make a new kind of cancer medicine. In May 2001, the drug Gleevec™ was approved to treat a rare cancer of the blood called chronic myelogenous leukemia (CML). The Food and Drug Administration described Gleevec's approval as "...a testament to the groundbreaking scientific research taking place in labs throughout America."

Researchers designed this drug to halt a cell-communication pathway that is always "on" in CML. Their success was founded on years of experiments in the basic biology of how cancer cells grow. The discovery of Gleevec is an example of the success of so-called molecular targeting: understanding how diseases arise at the level of cells, then figuring out ways to treat them. Scores of drugs, some to treat cancer but also many other health conditions, are in the research pipeline as a result of scientists' eavesdropping on how cells communicate.

出 典：©National Institute of General Medical Sciences, *Medicines By Design*, p.2, 40, http://publications.nigms.nih.gov/medbydesign/foreword.html, http://publications.nigms.nih.gov/medbydesign/chapter4.html（2010年12月1日現在）.

17・2 Reading Comprehension

▶ **Question**   Circle T (true) or F (false) for each statement.

対応 SBO
SBOs 2,3,4

1. In 2050 we can have tailor-made medicines. (　)

2. Today, if you and a friend have almost the same body size and age, you may get the same amount of a prescribed medicine. (　)

3. Genomics is the study of all of an organism's proteins. (　)

4. Although humans have 25,000 genes, each gene can cause thousands of different variations of the same protein. (　)

5. Gleevec, a tailor-made medicine for chronic myelogenous leukemia, works by halting a cell-communication pathway in patients with CML. (　)

17・3 Grammatical Rule: 挿入語句 (Parenthesis)

対応 SBO
SBOs 2,4,5

前後をカンマ，ダッシュ，またはカッコで区切り，付加的に加えられた情報を挿入語句という．挿入語句は意味的な関係は別として，前後の文とは文法的に独立している．

挿入語句には次のようなものがある．

(1) 注釈的な語句，文の挿入．

　　Although the idea that flavonols—*the bitter part of chocolate*—can help your cardiovascular health may have some merit, there's no strong scientific proof.

(2) 副詞節の挿入

　　How somebody looks at a situation, *whether they're a pessimist or optimist*, is likely to affect the outcome.

(3) 副詞句の挿入

　　BMI—*calculated by dividing weight in kilograms by height in meters squared*—is a standard way to determine how fat or thin a person is.

(4) I think や it seems などの挿入

　　The most interesting result of the study, *she says*, involved a hormone called leptin.

では，本文中の例文を見てみよう．挿入語句が文中でどのような働きをしているか考えてみよう．

> The science of pharmacology—*understanding the basics of how our bodies react to medicines and how medicines affect our bodies*—is already a vital part of 21st-century research.

17・4 Writing

対応 SBO
SBOs 5,8

警告に関する表現を学ぼう．

以下の表現は，危険や警告に関する形容詞である．それぞれを使って短い文をつくりなさい．

1. flammable 燃えやすい，引火性の
   エタノール（ethanol）は燃えやすいので注意するように．

   _____
   _____

2. toxic 毒性がある，有毒の
   この法律は有毒廃棄物（toxic waste）の処理（disposal）について規定している（regulate）．

   _____
   _____
   _____

3. explosive 爆発の，爆発
   工場で爆発事故があったが，幸い，放射線の脅威（radiological threat）は報告されていない．

   _____
   _____
   _____

17・5 Medical Vocabulary

対応 SBO
SBO 13

Write the Japanese expression of each of the following terms.

1. administration, medication　　　投　薬
2. by mouth, orally　　　経　口
3. by inhalation　　　_____
4. by rectum, rectally　　　_____
5. p.c.（= after meals）　　　_____
6. a.c.（= before meals）　　　_____
7. b.i.d.（= twice a day）　　　_____
8. t.i.d.（= three times a day）　　　_____

17 · 6 Listening/Speaking

対応 SBO
SBOs 11,12

CD Track 27

You will hear a short explanation about pharmacy practice. The explanation will not be printed in your textbook. You will hear the explanation only once, so you must listen carefully and answer in English. Be sure to answer the questions in full sentences.

1. What are common forms of medicines for children in Japan?

   _____

2. Do all medicines taste the same?

   _____

3. Who is this talk most likely directed towards?

   _____

Naturally Spoken English Notes:

your = yer   daughter = daughder   doctor = dacder

COLUMN

アドヒアランス（Adherence）

患者が処方どおり服薬できていることを"コンプライアンス（compliance；服薬遵守）が良好である"といい，飲み忘れなどにより規則正しく守れていない場合を"ノンコンプライアンス（non-compliance）"と表現してきた．しかし，この概念は患者を医療者の指示にどの程度従うかということで評価し，ノンコンプライアンスの原因は患者側にあるとすることから，近年では，"アドヒアランス（adherence）"という概念が重要視されてきている．

アドヒアランスとは，粘着，執着心を意味し，患者自身が積極的に治療方針の決定に参加し，相談のうえで決定した内容に従って治療を受けるという概念である．すなわち，医療者の指示に従順であるべきという患者像からさらに一歩進め，患者が主体となり，自分自身の医療に自ら責任をもって積極的に治療に取組む新たな患者像を目指すものである．

特に生活習慣病の治療などは，長期にわたって服薬の必要がある．患者の主体性が重要な領域では，服薬を妨げる因子などについて患者とともに考え，相談のうえで最適の治療法を決定していく．そうすることにより，良好な服薬アドヒアランスが得られ，治療成功が導かれる．

（木津純子）

Chapter 18

Nanotechnology and Drug Delivery

Objectives

After studying this chapter, you should be able to:

- Explain in English or Japanese what nanotechnology is and why it is important to make a "smart" drug. [SBO 2]
- Explain the content of English, including technical terms, related to pharmacy in Japanese or English. [SBO 3]
- Correctly explain English written for the sciences and related to clinical practice in Japanese or English. [SBO 4]
- Utilize one of the basic grammatical rules, nominal construction, for reading and writing. [SBOs 2, 4, 5]
- Rewrite short Japanese sentences into English without grammatical errors. [SBO 5]
- Write a self-introduction or letter in English. [SBO 6]
- List basic measurements, numbers, and phenomena related to the natural sciences in English. [SBO 7]
- Summarize the understood content of an English conversation between two pharmacy students. [SBO 11]
- Ask and answer questions that come up in an English conversation. [SBO 12]

対応 SBO
SBOs 2,3

18・1 Reading

先端技術の一分野であるナノテクノロジーは，原子や分子を操作することによって非常に小さい構造物をつくることができる．この技術は，薬が人体に入り，いくつもの障壁を乗り越えて，効果を発揮する目的の場所まで安全に運ばれることを可能にする．小さな精鋭たちの活躍を一緒にのぞいてみよう．

drug therapy
薬物治療〔療法〕

facet（物事の一つの）相，様相

drug delivery 薬物送達，ドラッグデリバリー

parenteral
（薬の投与が）非経口の

Drug therapy is a key facet of medical treatment for both acute and chronic diseases. The two most common methods of drug delivery used today are oral and parenteral (injection). Drugs taken orally are currently limited to small molecules because therapeutic agents based on large biological molecules, such as proteins, (e.g. insulin for the control of blood sugar), are degraded by the digestive system. However, drugs based on small molecules can be non-specific, high in toxicity, and low in bioavailability (rapidly cleared from the body). These factors can lead to significant side effects.

Research Advances

The emergence of nanotechnology—the branch of engineering that deals with things smaller than 100 nanometers—has opened a new era of design-driven research into the development of "smart" drug delivery systems. These delivery systems can potentially package highly potent drugs and target specific diseased tissues or cells while minimizing side effects.

Increasing Bioavailability

Drugs that are administered by injection are often cleared from the body before they reach or accumulate in the targeted tissues. Among the promising approaches to address this problem are the design and synthesis of new nanometer size drug carrier vehicles with surface structures that mimic those of native cells. These carriers allow the drug to remain in circulation by delaying or avoiding elimination or destruction by the body until the drug can accumulate in the targeted tissues.

Increasing Solubility

The solubility of hydrophobic, or poorly water soluble, drugs can be improved by impregnating these drugs in multi-layer nanoparticles with hydrophobic cores. The nanometer size of these particles also facilitates their uptake by cells because of the relative size differences (drug carrying nanoparticles can be 1000 times smaller than the target cell in diseased tissues).

18. Nanotechnology and Drug Delivery

Targeted Delivery

The ability to target the delivery of a therapeutic agent to a specific organ or tissue can greatly reduce side effects associated with systemic dosing. The new generation of designed nanoparticles can be labeled with targeting elements that attach to specific sites on the surface of cells and facilitate entry into the cell. One example is the attachment of ligands (bound molecules) to the surface of nanoparticles which confer the ability to bind specifically to receptors that are abundant only in targeted cells such as tumor cells for the delivery of anticancer agents or targeted tissues for gene therapy.

Protein Delivery

Proteins and other high molecular weight (macromolecular) biopolymers are an important class of therapeutic agents that are limited to intravenous or intramuscular injection due to degradation by stomach acid and enzymes in the digestive tract. The ability to deliver these molecules intact orally would have a high impact on the treatment of diseases such as type 1 diabetes which currently requires intramuscular injection of insulin. One approach utilizes bioresponsive polymers as drug carriers that can change shape in response to the acidity of the surrounding environment. These new materials shield acid sensitive drugs during passage through the stomach and can selectively attach and deliver their payloads to the mucosal lining of the small intestine for release into the blood stream. These types of approaches may enable the full potential of protein based drugs for the treatment of diseases in the near future.

出 典: Elias A. Zerhouni, M.D. "National Institute of Biomedical Imaging and Bioengineering Five-Year Professional Judgment Budget", National Institute of Biomedical Imaging and Bioengineering, Department of Health and Human Services, National Institute of Health, p.12～13 (2005), www.nibib.nih.gov/nibib/file/AboutNIBIB/BudgetandLegislation/FY2006/NIBIBHouseFY2006.pdf-02-24-2009 (2009年12月20日現在).

18・2 Reading Comprehension

▶ **Question**　Answer the following questions in English.

対応 SBO
SBOs 2,3,4

1. What are the two most common ways of drug delivery used today?

   _____

2. What factors of drugs, based on small molecules, can cause serious side effects?

   _____

3. What is one of the promising approaches to address the problem with parenteral drugs?

   _____

4. What advantage can targeted delivery bring?

   _____

5. What treatment would be greatly influenced by orally delivering large molecule therapeutic agents intact?

   _____

   _____

18・3　Grammatical Rule: 名詞構文 (Nominal Construction)

対応 SBO
SBOs 2,4,5

　英語表現の特色の一つに名詞構文がある．名詞構文とは"動詞または形容詞が名詞化されて文に組込まれた構文"である．この表現は，冗長な文を簡明に表現できることが長所であり，自然科学の英文によくみられる．

　名詞構文には次のようなものがある．

(1) 元の語が自動詞の場合

　　You will live happily → your happy life

(2) 元の語が他動詞の場合

　　He loves science deeply → his deep love of science

(3) 元の語が形容詞の場合

　　I am certain that he is honest → my certainty of his honesty

　上記の(2)では，誰が love なのか，何を love なのかを見失ってはならない．つまり，必ず意味上の主語と目的語が何であるか，また，後続する前置詞句があった場合には，前置詞句と名詞との意味関係をしっかり考えて解釈することが大切である．

　では，本文中の例文を見てみよう．イタリックの名詞構文の意味関係を考えてみよう．

> One example is *the attachment of ligands to the surface of nanoparticles ...*

18. Nanotechnology and Drug Delivery

対応 SBO
SBOs 5,6

18・4 Writing

英文 E メール(1) ── 件名と書き出し（呼びかけ）

例）件名（Subject）：Questions about the research grant
呼びかけと書き出し：
Dear Sir or Madam,（相手の名前がわからないとき）
My name is Hanako Yakugaku and I am a third-year student at ABC University. I would like to ask some questions about the research grant offered by your foundation.

例を参考に，次の状況設定で，件名とメール本文の書き出しを考えてみよう．

件名：奨学金の申し込みについて

_____

_____

呼びかけと書き出し：掲示版に張ってあった奨学金について，いつ申し込んだら よいかを質問する．係の名前は不明．

_____
_____
_____
_____
_____
_____
_____
_____
_____

対応 SBO
SBO 7

18・5 Medical Vocabulary

Write a word for each of the following abbreviations.

1. cm   (centimeter)   2. mm   (   )
3. μm   (micrometer)   4. kg   (   )
5. mg   (   )   6. μg, mcg (   )
7. L   (liter   )   8. dL   (   )
9. mL   (   )   10. μL   (   )

18·6 Listening / Speaking

You will hear a short conversation between two people. The conversation will not be printed in your textbook. You will hear the conversation only once, so you must listen carefully and answer the questions in English. Be sure to answer the questions in full sentences.

対応 SBO
SBOs 11,12
Track 28

1. Where did this conversation most likely take place?

   _____

2. What was the homework?

   _____

3. Why should the students summarize the readings?

   _____

Naturally Spoken English Notes:

would you = woudja   have to = hafta

COLUMN

1回飲むだけで1週間有効，1回の注射で3カ月間有効！

最近はナノ（10^{-9} m）粒子が注目されているが，粒子径が数マイクロ（10^{-6} m）程度の球状の製剤である**マイクロスフェア**はすでに医薬品に応用され，薬の有効性を高め，患者の負担を減らす役割を果たしている．マイクロスフェアとは，高分子でできた三次元の網目構造の球状粒子中に薬物を分散させたものである．たとえば，アジスロマイシンという抗菌薬をマイクロスフェアの中に分散した製剤は，たった1回の服用で感染症の治療に有効である．また前立腺癌や閉経前乳癌の治療に使用されるリュープロレリンは，マイクロスフェアに入れて皮下注射すると，12週間にわたってリュープロレリンが持続的に放出される．皮下注射されたマイクロスフェアが徐々に体内で分解されることにより，中に閉じ込められていた薬が徐々に放出されるのである．また，マイクロスフェアは生体内で分解される高分子を用いており，皮下投与しても安全である．このように，マイクロスフェアの技術が医薬品の有効性と安全性を高める目的で活用されている．今後，**ナノスフェア**の技術が医療応用されることにより，どのような機能をもった医薬品製剤が誕生してくるかとても楽しみである．

(中村明弘)

Chapter 19

Inside Clinical Trials: Testing Medical Products in People

Objectives

After studying this chapter, you should be able to:

- Read simple written sentences and identify the main idea in a timely fashion. [SBO 1]
- Explain the content of simple written passages in Japanese or English. [SBO 2]
- Explain in English or Japanese what clinical trials are and how they proceed. [SBO 3]
- Correctly explain English written for the sciences and related to clinical practice in Japanese or English. [SBO 4]
- Utilize one of the basic grammatical rules, concord, for reading and writing. [SBOs 2, 4, 5]
- Rewrite short Japanese sentences about campus life into English without grammatical errors. [SBO 5]
- Write a self-introduction or letter in English. [SBO 6]
- Explain the content of English, including technical terms, related to pharmacy in Japanese or English. [SBO 3]
- Summarize the understood content of an English conversation. [SBO 11]
- Answer the questions about a short announcement on pharmaceutical education in English. [SBO 12]
- Correctly pronounce the names of illnesses, parts of the body, and drugs. [SBO 13]

対応 SBO
SBOs 1,2,3,4

19・1 Reading

治験（臨床試験）という言葉は，最近新聞でもよく目にするようになってきた．それは動物実験の次の段階としてヒトに行われる試験のようだ．薬が認可される前に必ず必要だというが，具体的にはどのようなステップで進められていくのだろうか．一緒に見ていこう．

What Happens in a Clinical Trial?

Every clinical trial is carefully designed to answer certain research questions. A trial plan called a protocol maps out what study procedures will be done, by whom, and why.

The clinical trial team includes doctors and nurses, as well as other health care professionals. This team checks the health of the participant at the beginning of the trial and assesses whether that person is eligible to participate. Those found to be eligible—and who agree to participate—are given specific instructions, and then monitored and carefully assessed during the trial and after it is completed.

Done at hospitals and research centers around the country, clinical trials are conducted in phases. Phase 1 trials try to determine dosing, document how a drug is metabolized and excreted, and identify acute side effects. Usually, a small number of healthy volunteers (between 20 and 80) are used in Phase 1 trials.

Phase 2 trials include more participants (about 100-300) who have the disease or condition that the product potentially could treat. In Phase 2 trials, researchers seek to gather further safety data and preliminary evidence of the drug's beneficial effects (efficacy), and they develop and refine research methods for future trials with this drug. If the Phase 2 trials indicate that the drug may be effective—and the risks are considered acceptable, given the observed efficacy and the severity of the disease—the drug moves to Phase 3.

In Phase 3 trials, the drug is studied in a larger number of people with the disease (approximately 1,000-3,000). This phase further tests the product's effectiveness, monitors side effects and, in some cases, compares the product's effects to a standard treatment, if one is already available.

Phase 2 and Phase 3 clinical trials generally involve a "control" standard. In many studies, one group of volunteers will be given an experimental or "test" drug or treatment, while the control group is given either a standard treatment for the illness or an inactive pill, liquid, or powder that has no treatment value (placebo). This control group provides a basis for comparison for assessing effects of the test treatment. In some studies, the control group will receive a placebo instead of an active drug or treatment. In other cases, it is considered unethical to use placebos, particularly if an effective treatment is available. Withholding treatment (even for a short time) would subject research participants to unreasonable risks.

The treatment each trial participant receives is often decided by a process called randomization. This process can be compared to a coin toss that is done by computer. During clinical trials, no one likely knows which therapy is better, and randomization assures that treatment selection will be free of any preference a physician may have. Randomization increases the likelihood that the groups of people receiving the test drug or control are comparable at the start of the trial, enabling comparisons in health status between groups of patients who participated in the trial.

In conjunction with randomization, a feature known as blinding helps ensure that bias doesn't distort the conduct of a trial or the interpretation of its results. Single-blinding means the participant does not know whether he or she is receiving the experimental drug, an established treatment for that disease, or a placebo. In a single-blinded trial, the research team does know what the participant is receiving.

A double-blinded trial means that neither the participant nor the research team knows during the trial which participants receive the experimental drug. The patient will usually find out what he or she received at a pre-specified time in the trial.

出 典： © U.S. Food and Drug Administration, "Inside Clinical Trials: Testing Medical Products in People", http://www.fda.gov/Drugs/ResourcesForYou/Consumers/ucm143531.htm (2010年12月1日現在).

19・2　Reading Comprehension

本文中で使われている次の治験用語に相当する日本語の用語を（　）内に記入し，下の (a)〜(g) から定義を選んで記号を [　] 内に記入しなさい．

対応 SBO
SBOs 2,3,4

1. double-blinded trial　（　　　　　　　）［　］
2. effectiveness　　　　（　　　　　　　）［　］
3. efficacy　　　　　　（　　　　　　　）［　］
4. eligible　　　　　　（　　　　　　　）［　］
5. placebo　　　　　　（　　　　　　　）［　］
6. protocol　　　　　　（　　　　　　　）［　］
7. randomization　　　（　　　　　　　）［　］

a. an inactive substance or procedure designed to resemble the test treatment
b. a method to assign participants to study groups based on chance
c. a clinical trial design in which neither the participants nor the study staff knows what treatment the participants are receiving
d. the typical effect of a medical product in regular use
e. a written plan for a clinical trial
f. meeting the criteria for entry into a clinical trial
g. the degree to which a medical product produces a desired result under the idealized circumstances of a clinical trial

19・3　Grammatical Rule：数の呼応（Concord）

対応 SBO
SBOs 2,4,5

動詞の数（単・複）は，主語が単数であるか，複数であるかによって決まる．これを"呼応"，または"数の一致"とよぶ．英語を書く際に，以下の点に留意することが大切である．

(1) 主語が both 〜 and... で結ばれたとき，動詞は複数形になる．
　　Both you and I *are* anxious to study English.
(2) and で結ばれた主語が，every, each で始まるとき，動詞は単数形になる．
　　Every student and professor *has* to join this tour.
(3) There is 構文で，主語である最初の名詞句が単数のとき，動詞は単数形になる．
　　There *is* a lot of hospitality and personal care in this hospital.
(4) 主語が or, nor, either 〜 or ..., neither 〜 nor ..., not only 〜 but (also) ... で結ばれているとき，動詞の数は動詞に最も近い名詞に呼応する（近接呼応）．
　　Not only you but also I *am* to blame.
(5) more than ＋単数名詞，half of ＋単数名詞のとき，動詞は単数になり，more than ＋複数名詞，half of ＋複数名詞のときは，動詞は複数で呼応する．
　　More than one professor *is* taking care of the student.
(6) as well as, (together) with, no less than などが用いられた主語は，形式的な英語では，通例，前後にカンマをつけ，動詞との数の呼応に影響しない．ただし，略式的な英語では，前後にカンマをつけず，動詞の呼応に影響することがある．
　　That student, as well as his friends, *is* to blame.　（形式的）
　　That student as well as his friends *are* to blame.　（略式的）

19. Inside Clinical Trials: Testing Medical Products in People

では，本文中の下記の例文を見てみよう．（　）内の動詞はどのように呼応するか考えてみよう．

> A double-blinded trial means that *neither* the participant *nor* the research team (know) during the trial which participants receive the experimental drug.

19・4 Writing

対応 SBO
SBOs 5,6

英文 E メール(2) —— 本文のまとめと終わり方（結句）

例）Please let me know if I can see you at 5:00PM tomorrow to discuss the matter.
　　Sincerely yours,
　　Hanako

これを例に，下記のまとめと結句を英語で書いてみよう．

　応募用紙を昨日郵送いたしました．金曜日までに着かない場合，お知らせいただけるとありがたいのですが．
敬具
（自分の名前）

_____

_____

_____

_____

_____

_____

19・5 Medical Vocabulary

対応 SBO
SBOs 3,13

Match the terms with their definitions and write the appropriate letter (a～e) to the right of each term.

1. adenitis　　（　　）　　a. any muscle disease

2. diarrhea　　（　　）　　b. pain in the stomach

3. gastralgia　（　　）　　c. frequent passage of watery stool

4. myopathy　 （　　）　　d. tumor of immature cells

5. blastoma　　（　　）　　e. inflammation of a gland

19. Inside Clinical Trials: Testing Medical Products in People

19・6 Listening/Speaking

対応 SBO
SBOs 11,12
Track 29

You will hear a short announcement about pharmaceutical education. The announcement will not be printed in your textbook. You will hear the announcement only once, so you must listen carefully and answer in English. Be sure to answer the questions in full sentences.

1. Is attending the talk optional?

   _____

2. What is the theme of the presentation?

   _____

3. After the talk, what will the participants do?

   _____

Naturally Spoken English Notes:

   strategies = stradegies   communicating = communicading
   going to = gonna

COLUMN

治験とは

　化学合成や，植物，土壌中，海洋生物などから発見された物質のなかから，動物実験などにより，病気に効果があり，人に使用しても安全と予測されるものが"くすりの候補"として選ばれる．この"くすりの候補"の開発の最終段階では，健康な人や患者の協力によって，ヒトでの効果と安全性を調べる．こうして得られた成績を国が審査して，病気の治療に必要で，かつ安全に使っていけると認められたものが"くすり"となる．ヒトで行う研究を"臨床試験"という．"くすりの候補"を用いて国の承認を得るために，安全でヒトに役立つかどうかを確認するための臨床試験のことを特に"治験"とよぶ．従来，承認を得ることが目的であったため"治験"は企業主導で行われてきたが，薬事法が改正され必ずしも企業の開発プロセスにのる必要はなく医師主導での実施も可能となった．ただ，小児では倫理上の問題などから臨床試験を実施することが難しいため，小児用の医薬品開発は進んでいないのが現状である．実際，小児で使用される医薬品の3/4はその添付文書に小児での用法・用量の明確な記載がない．

（入倉　充）

Chapter 20

Self-Medication

Objectives

After studying this chapter, you should be able to:

- Read simple written sentences and identify the main idea in a timely fashion. [SBO 1]
- Explain the content of simple written passages in Japanese or English. [SBO 2]
- Explain in English or Japanese what self-medication is and why it is important for ourselves and society. [SBO 3]
- Correctly explain English written for the sciences and related to clinical practice in Japanese or English. [SBO 4]
- Utilize one of the basic grammatical rules, clause, for reading and writing. [SBOs 2, 4, 5]
- Rewrite short Japanese sentences about Japanese culture and campus life into English without grammatical errors. [SBO 5]
- Write a self-introduction or letter in English. [SBO 6]
- Explain the content of English, including technical terms, related to pharmacy in Japanese or English. [SBO 3]
- Tell the difference between sounds in spoken English. [SBO 10]
- Summarize the understood content of an English conversation. [SBO 11]
- Ask and answer questions that come up in an English conversation between two pharmacy students. [SBO 12]
- Correctly pronounce the names of illnesses, parts of the body, and drugs. [SBO 13]

対応 SBO
SBOs 1,2,3,4

20・1 Reading

> 今日のわが国は，少子高齢化，医師不足，医療費負担の増大，生活習慣病の増加といった問題に直面している．同時に，IT化の進歩に伴い，病気に関する情報は正しいか否かにかかわらずあふれている．セルフメディケーションとは，医師の相談なしに，患者自らの判断で，軽いケガや病気の手当てを自分で行うことである．そのためには，患者は正しい情報と的確な判断が必要になり，薬のプロとしての薬剤師のアドバイスは，登録販売員とは一線を画す重要なより所となろう．

Self-medication is the treatment of common health problems with medicines especially designed and labeled for use without medical supervision and approved as safe and effective for such use.

Society and Public Health

Society benefits from a citizenry that is better informed about healthcare and therefore more able to exercise self-reliance. Having the tools available to help consumers practice such self-reliance also allows scarce health resources to be directed toward illnesses or conditions that require treatment in the professional healthcare system. Having appropriate nonprescription medicines available can also reduce illegal use of prescription products without a prescription—something which occurs too frequently in some countries, and is sometimes referred to as "self-prescription." In Mexico, for example, an increase in the availability of nonprescription medicines helped to reduce the estimated rate of "self-prescription" by 20 percent from 1989 to 1999.

Government and Health Professional Outlooks

Many national and international organizations have looked at how best to establish and structure national drug policies within their healthcare systems. As a starting point, one fundamental to keep in mind was articulated at an International Conference on Primary Health Care, held in Alma-Ata in 1978:

"People have the right and duty to participate individually and collectively in the planning and implementation of their health care."

In line with a philosophy of individual participation and empowerment, the World Health Organization has stated that responsible self-medication can:

- Help prevent and treat symptoms and ailments that do not require medical consultation;
- Reduce the increasing pressure on medical services for the relief of

minor ailments, especially when financial and human resources are limited;

- Increase the availability of health care to populations living in rural or remote areas where access to medical advice may be difficult; and
- Enable patients to control their own chronic conditions.

As the most accessible form of health care, self-medication fills a series of valuable and sometimes crucial functions for individuals and healthcare systems. That healthcare systems as well as individuals benefit from self-medication emphasizes the need for clear policies by national governments. Those policies should recognize the positive role played by products specifically intended for self-medication and should meet their citizens' desires to take an active role in their health. As a US Commissioner of Food and Drugs noted:

"The Food and Drug Administration accepts the concept of self-medication. The consumer demands it; the law provides for it; and it is in fact a vital part of our nation's health care system."

In Europe, the European Parliament stated that it:

"Considers that responsible self-medication should be further promoted, which will foster the growing desire of the European Union's citizens to take responsibility for their own health and also help reduce health expenditure. In recent years, responsible self-medication has been identified as an important element in long term health policy by the institutions of the European Community."

Health professional organizations have also drawn attention to the importance of self-medication. The World Medical Association, for example, published a statement on self-medication in 2002, drawing attention to some of the themes in this publication—the importance of a clear prescription-nonprescription distinction and the role and importance of labeling for safe and effective use, as well as guidance for physicians and their patients regarding responsible self-medication. The International Pharmaceutical Federation adopted a joint statement on self-medication with WSMI to highlight the common goals of our two groups: to provide high quality service to the public and to encourage the responsible use of medicines.

The International Pharmaceutical Federation 国際薬学連合

WSMI (= The World Self-Medication Industry) 世界セルフメディケーション協会

出典：© World Self-Medication Industry, http://www.wsmi.org/aboutsm.htm （2010年12月1日現在）.

20・2 Reading Comprehension

▶ **Question**　Based on the reading passage, put either T (true) or F (false) in the parentheses for each statement.

1. Self-medication is the treatment of chronic illness with OTC or prescription drugs by individual patients.　　（　　）
2. Self-prescription is the illegitimate use of prescription drugs without medical consultation.　　（　　）
3. The WHO has reported that self-medication is useful for people living in inaccessible areas.　　（　　）
4. The European Parliament thinks self-medication is good for the poor to cut down on their expenditures.　　（　　）
5. The goals of the International Pharmaceutical Federation are to provide high quality service to the public and to recommend careful use of medicines with responsibility.　　（　　）

対応 SBO
SBOs 2,3,4

20・3 Grammatical Rule：節（Clause）

節（clause）とは，"接続詞・関係詞＋主語＋動詞"から成る語の集まりをいう．節は，文中では名詞，形容詞，副詞の働きをし，それに応じて名詞節，形容詞節，副詞節とよばれる．

(1) 名詞節（that, whether などの接続詞に導かれ，文の主語，動詞の目的語，動詞の補語，前置詞の目的語，直前の名詞の内容を説明する同格として働く．）
　　I hope *that your study of organic chemistry will be fruitful*.
(2) 形容詞節（関係代名詞・関係副詞に導かれ，先行する名詞を後ろから修飾する．）
　　God helps those *who help themselves*.
(3) 副詞節（従属接続詞 when, because, if などに導かれ，主節（中の動詞）を修飾し，時，原因，理由，条件，譲歩，目的，結果，様態などを表す．）
　　You don't realize the value of friendship *until you lose it*.

では，本文中の次の例文を見てみよう．下線部は何節か，どのような働きをしているか考えてみよう．

対応 SBO
SBOs 2,4,5

> Having the tools available to help consumers practice such self-reliance also allows scarce health resources to be directed toward illnesses or conditions <u>that require treatment in the professional healthcare system.</u>

20・4 Writing

英文 E メール (3) —— メール文の校正

作文の後，読み直して推敲(すいこう)することは英語でも必要不可欠なステップである．大学の交換留学生である Andrew Chen に英語を習おうと思い，次のメール文を書いてみた．文法上の間違いや，文のつなぎ方，あるいは表現や丁寧さの度合いが不適切なところを指摘し，正しく書き直しなさい．訂正が必要な個所は 8 カ所ある．

Dear Mr. Andrew,
I want to practice English conversation, but I don't have many chance to do so. If you are not too busy on weekends, would you teach me English? I am convenient on Saturday afternoon. Although I live near the station, I can see you at the coffee shop in front of the station. Please respond to me.
Yours faithfully,
Takahashi

20・5 Medical Vocabulary

Write the name of each numbered part on the corresponding line.

(1) 表 皮 _____

(2) 真 皮 _____

(3) 毛 _____

(4) 脂 腺 _____

(5) 汗 腺 _____

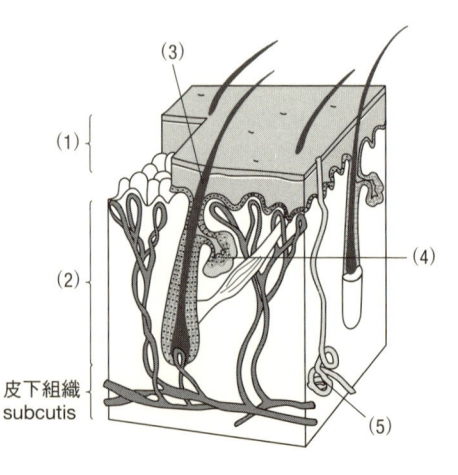

20・6 Listening/Speaking

You will hear a short conversation. The conversation will not be printed in your textbook. You will hear the conversation only once, so you must listen carefully and answer in English. Be sure to answer the questions in full sentences.

対応 SBO
SBOs 10,11,12,13
Track 30

1. Why didn't Shinichi see Chris for a long time?

2. What were Chris's symptoms?

3. Did the doctor prescribe any medicine?

4. Basically, what did Chris do all last week?

COLUMN

医薬分業の意義,セルフメディケーション

　医薬分業とは医師と薬剤師がお互いの専門性を独立させ,お互いの職能を尊重しながらよりよい薬物療法を提供することである.1974年が日本の分業元年といわれ,医師の処方せん料が大幅に引き上げられ,医薬分業が誘導された.医薬分業のメリットとして,薬剤師による二重鑑査や院内在庫にかかわりなく自由に薬剤を選択できる,薬価差益による"薬漬け"からの解放,処方の公開による医療の公開の進展などがある.

　セルフメディケーションとは,"自己の健康管理のため,医薬品などを自分の意思で使用することである.薬剤師は生活者に対し,医薬品などについて情報を提供し,アドバイスする役割を担う"(日本薬剤師会)と定義している.セルフメディケーションを広義でとらえると医療だけでなく看護,介護,食生活,運動などさまざまな分野が関係してくるが,おもにはOTC薬の使用が中心であり薬剤師が積極的にかかわる必要がある.

(上村直樹)

Appendix

1. 発音ルール表
2. 発音記号（phonetic symbol）一覧表
3. ライティングのヒント

Appendix 1. 発音ルール表

		ア	イ	ウ	エ	オ
短母音	æ	短くて強勢のあるa				
	ʌ	o, u, (ou) でアと読むとき (前後にm, n, u など)	i, y	u, (-ook)	e, (ea)	o, (w+)a
	ə	弱音節で				
長母音	ɑː	ar, a (+l, ff, ss, f, s, n など)	iː e, ee, ea, ie, ei, i	uː oo, (u)		
	əː	ir, ur, er, (our), (w+)or				ɔː au, aw, or, al, (ough+t)
二重母音	ou	ou, ow			ei a, ai, ay, (ei, ey)	ou o, oa, (ou, ow)
	ai	i, y			ɛə air, ear, are, ere	ɔi oi, oy
			ia eer, ear, ere	uə ure, oor		(ɔə) or, oor

分節のルール
1. 長母音, 二重母音/子音 pa/per
2. 子音+強勢のある短母音/子音+強勢のある短母音+子音母音/子音 ri/ver doc/tor
3. 弱母音 be/low
4. [l, m, n] は音節子音 bot/tle, sud/den
5. 複合語, 合成語は構成要素に分け, 各構成要素を音節に分ける un/think/ing/ly back/bone

進行同化 progressive assimilation AB>AA twenty [tweni]
逆行同化 regressive assimilation AB>BB I can go [ai kəŋ gou]
融合同化 coalescent assimilation AB>C miss you [mɪʃ uː]

		強形	弱形		強形	弱形		強形	弱形
	a	[ei]	[ə]	may	[mei]	[me, mi, me]	that	[ðæt]	[ðət]
	the	[ðiː]	[ði, ðə, ð]	must	[mʌst]	[məst, mes, mst, ms]	some	[sʌm]	[səm, sm]
	am	[æm]	[əm, m]	shall	[ʃæl]	[ʃəl, ʃl, əl, ʃə, ʃ, l]	but	[bʌt]	[bət, bt]
	are	[ɑːr]	[ər, r]	will	[wil]	[wəl, əl, l]	by	[bai]	[bəi, bə, bi]
	was	[wɔz]	[wəz, wz]	should	[ʃud]	[ʃəd, ʃd, ʃt, d]	for	[fɔːr]	[fər, fr]
	were	[wəːr]	[wər]	would	[wud]	[wəd, əd, d]	from	[frəm]	[frəm, frm]
	can	[kæn]	[kən, kn, kŋ]	he	[hiː]	[hi, iː, i]	of	[ɑv]	[əv, v]
	could	[kud]	[kəd, kd, kt]	him	[him]	[im, əm]	to	[tuː]	[tu+母音, tə+子音]
	do	[duː]	[du, də, d]	she	[ʃiː]	[ʃi]	and	[ænd]	[ənd, ən, nd, n]
	does	[dʌz]	[dəz, dəs, dz]	her	[həːr]	[hər, ər]	there	[ðɛər]	[ðər]
	has	[hæz]	[həz, əz, z, s]	us	[ʌs]	[əs, s]	till	[til]	[tl]
	have	[hæv]	[həv, əv, v, f]	they	[ðei]	[ðe, ði]	what	[hwɑt]	[hwət]
				them	[ðem]	[ðəm, ðm, əm]	who	[huː]	[hu, u, u]

	強形	弱形
ng→[ŋ]	have to [hæv tuː]	[hæftə]
	has to [hæz tuː]	[hæstə]
th [θ] [ð] その他有声音	used to [juːst tuː]	[juːstə]
sh→[ʃ]	ought to [ɔːt tuː]	[ɔːtə]
ch, tch→[tʃ]	want to [wɑnt tuː]	[wɑnə]
dge, j [dʒ]	going to [gouiŋ tuː]	[gənə]
g+e, i	verb-ing [-iŋ]	[-in]
	pretty [priti]	[prəti] (adv.)
	Saint, St [seint]	[sənt, sən, sin, sn]

Appendix 2. 発音記号（phonetic symbol）一覧表

発音記号	つづり字例	発音記号	つづり字例
母　音			
[iː]/[i]†1	s*ea*t	[ɔ]/Am.[ɒ]	f*o*x
[i]/[ɪ]†1	s*i*t	[ʌ]	*u*nder
[e]/[ɛ]†1	s*e*t	[əː]	*ea*rly
[æ]	s*a*t	[ə]	*a*bove
[ɑː]	f*a*ther	[uː]	p*oo*l
[ɔː]	*a*ll	[u]/[ʊ]†1	p*u*ll
二重母音			
[ei]	*a*ce	[iə]/[iɚ]†2	*ear*
[ai]	*eye*	[ɛə]/[ɛɚ]†2	*air*
[ɔi]	b*oy*	[ɔə]/[ɔɚ]†2	d*oor*
[au]	*ou*t	[uə]/[uɚ]†2	p*oor*
[ou]/Br.[əu]	h*o*me		
子　音			
[p]	*p*en	[k]	*k*ey
[b]	*b*ook	[g]	*g*ood
[t]	*t*ea	[f]	*f*ish
[d]	*d*esk	[v]	*v*ery
[θ]	*th*ink	[l]	*l*ook
[ð]	*th*ere	[tʃ]	*ch*urch
[s]	*s*ink	[dʒ]	*J*apan
[z]	*z*ink	[m]	*m*ouse
[ʃ]	*sh*ip	[n]	*n*urse
[ʒ]	vi*s*ion	[ŋ]	si*ng*
[h]	*h*ot	[w]	*w*ool
[r]	*r*ice	[j]	*y*et

†1　辞書によって表記法が異なる場合がある．
†2　Br.E. では語末の [r] は発音せず，Am.E. では巻き舌で発音する．

Appendix 3. ライティングのヒント

1. はじめに

大学におけるライティングとは，和文英訳というよりむしろ，自分の考えや伝えたいことを英語で表現するということに重点が置かれます．難しい，自信がない，と思う人がいるかもしれませんが，自分の考えや意思を表現するよい機会だと思って練習してみてください．答えは一つではなく，いろいろなやり方がありますので，楽しんで英文をつくってみてください．

2. ライティングの流れ

"書く"という行為には次の3段階のステップが含まれます．

Step 1: 構想を練る（Brainstorming）

まず自分は何を言いたいのか，日本語でよいのでよく考えてみてください．しっかりした構想なしに書き始めると，途中でつぎに何を書いたらよいかわからなくなってしまいます．

Step 2: 実際に書いてみる（First Draft）

英文を考えるのに和英辞書を使う場合には，最初に記載されている単語をすぐに使うのではなく，どの英語がぴったりするか注意して選んでください．わからないときには，さらに英和辞典や英英辞典を使うとよいでしょう．

Step 3: 読み返してみて推敲する（Editing）

皆さんは日本語で何か書くとき，いったん書き終えたら，その後自分の書いたものを読み直すと思いますが，英語でも同じです．ほかの人が読んで理解できるかどうかを意識しながら読み返し，必要に応じて推敲しましょう．文の構成，単語の選び方，文法，スペルをチェックしましょう．

3. Eメールの書き方

ここでは，携帯のメール（text message）ではなく，パソコンのアドレスから送るEメールの書き方について基本的な注意事項を述べます．たとえば皆さんが，大学の外国人の先生や留学生と連絡をとる際には，どのようにしたらよいでしょうか．

a. 件名を忘れずに！

件名がない，あるいは適切でない場合，迷惑メールと間違えられたり，読んでもらえなかったりする可能性があります．簡潔に，かつ適切に内容を表す件名をつけましょう．

良い例: Assignment of French Class

悪い例: Hello（内容が何かわからない）

b. 呼びかけも大事

つぎに相手に呼びかけます．先生の場合にはProfessorをつけるのが無難でしょう．会ったことがない人や仕事上の付き合いでは，Mr. Ms. などをつけます．友人や家族はファーストネームで呼びかけます．

良い例: Dear Professor Gunderson,

良い例：Dear Mrs. Hall,
　　悪い例：Dear Mr. Hiroshi,（ファーストネームに Mr. はつけない）
c. 必要に応じて簡単に自分の紹介をする.
　初めて連絡する場合や，大学の授業に関して連絡する場合には，簡単に自己紹介をします．
　　良い例：I am taking your microbiology class on Wednesdays.
　　良い例：I am a first-year student in the chorus club.
　　悪い例：Can I ask about the homework?（どの授業の宿題のことかわからない）
d. 用件を簡潔に，しかし丁寧に述べる.
　用件を的確に，簡潔に述べます．相手が先生の場合や，仕事上の連絡の場合には，失礼にならないように丁寧な表現を用いるようにしましょう．
　　良い例：I have a question about the lab report, and I wonder if I can see you some time next week.
　　良い例：I am grateful for all the help you gave me during my stay in your country.
　　悪い例：I could not understand the physics problem in the last class. When can you see me to explain it?（押しつけがましい）
　　悪い例：I have to go to the dentist tomorrow. Please reschedule our meeting.（命令調で相手によっては失礼になる）
e. 結びのことば
　状況に応じて，最後に一言，結びの言葉を書きます．
　　良い例：Your help would be appreciated.
　　良い例：Please give my best regards to Professor Tanaka.
　　悪い例：See you later.（メールでは使わない表現）
f. 挨拶と署名
　最初に簡単に自己紹介した場合にも，必ず最後に挨拶と名前を書いてください．挨拶は，丁寧な言い方として，Yours truly, Yours sincerely, Best regards, などがあり，一般的な言い方として Regards, というような表現があります．何かを依頼したり，お世話になったりした際には感謝の意を表す意味で Yours appreciatively, が使われます．また，署名はメールソフトで自動署名を設定しておくという方法もあります．
　　良い例：Yours sincerely,
　　　　　　　Misako Suzuki
　　悪い例：Regards, Atsushi Nakata（挨拶と署名が同じ行になっている）
以上のことに留意して，効果的なメールを書くようにしましょう．

第 1 版 第 1 刷 2011 年 2 月 2 日 発行
第 4 刷 2013 年 12 月 1 日 発行

プライマリー薬学シリーズ 1
薬 学 英 語 入 門

編　集　　公益社団法人 日本薬学会
Ⓒ2011　発行者　小 澤 美 奈 子
発　行　　株式会社 東京化学同人
東京都文京区千石 3 丁目36-7 (✆112-0011)
電話　03-3946-5311・FAX　03-3946-5316
URL: http://www.tkd-pbl.com/

印刷 中央印刷株式会社・製本 株式会社 青木製本所

ISBN 978-4-8079-1651-1　Printed in Japan
無断転載および複製物（コピー，電子
データなど）の配布，配信を禁じます．

実践的な薬学英会話集

薬学生・薬剤師のための
英会話ハンドブック

原　博・Eric M. Skier・渡辺朋子　著
新書判　2色刷　224ページ　定価3000円＋税　**CD付**

薬局や病院で薬剤師が，英語圏の患者に対応するときに役立つ実践的な英会話集．OTC薬の販売，受診勧告，服薬指導，病棟での治療薬の説明など実際の場面に沿った会話例を豊富に収載．ネイティブスピーカーにより主要スキットを録音した付録CDは，発音練習に役立つ．

2013年12月現在

日本薬学会 編
プライマリー薬学シリーズ
全5巻6冊
B5判・2色刷（第1巻は1色）・各巻約150ページ

"スタンダード薬学シリーズ"の学習に必要な
薬学準備教育のための教科書シリーズ

1 薬学英語入門 CD付
定価：本体 2800 円＋税

編集担当：入江徹美・金子利雄・河野　円・Eric M. Skier
竹内典子・中村明弘・堀内正子

2 薬学の基礎としての 物理学
定価：本体 2400 円＋税

編集担当：小澤俊彦・鈴木　巖・須田晃治・山岡由美子

3 薬学の基礎としての 化 学
Ⅰ．定量的取扱い
定価：本体 2400 円＋税

編集担当：小澤俊彦・鈴木　巖・須田晃治・山岡由美子

Ⅱ．有機化学
定価：本体 2400 円＋税

編集担当：石﨑　幸・伊藤　喬・原　博

4 薬学の基礎としての 生物学
定価：本体 2400 円＋税

編集担当：青木　隆・小宮山忠純・笹津備規

5 薬学の基礎としての 数学・統計学
定価：本体 2400 円＋税

編集担当：小澤俊彦・鈴木　巖・須田晃治・山岡由美子

2013 年 12 月現在

日本薬学会編
スタンダード薬学シリーズ
全11巻・24冊

```
――― シリーズ編集委員会 ―――
総 監 修  市 川  厚・工 藤 一 郎
編集委員長  長 野 哲 雄
副 委 員 長  入 江 徹 美・原    博
編 集 委 員  赤 池 昭 紀・笹 津 備 規
         須 田 晃 治・永 沼  章
```

領域編集担当

|1| ヒューマニズム・薬学入門
4200円
市川 厚・入江徹美・木内祐二
工藤一郎・中島宏昭・原 博

|2| 物理系薬学
佐治英郎・須田晃治・長野哲雄
本間 浩・勝 孝・中西 守・新津 勝
- I．物質の物理的性質（第2版）4400円
- II．化学物質の分析（第3版）3600円
- III．生体分子・化学物質の構造決定 3400円
- IV．演習編 勝 孝・金澤秀子・須田晃治・中垣良一・本間 浩 4000円

|3| 化学系薬学
伊藤 喬・長野哲雄・夏苅英昭・原 博
増野匡彦・佐藤雅之・竹谷孝一・鳥居塚和生
- I．化学物質の性質と反応（第2版）4900円
- II．ターゲット分子の合成と生体分子・医薬品の化学
3600円
- III．自然が生み出す薬物 4200円
- IV．演習編 伊藤 喬・原 博・増野匡彦 3200円

|4| 生物系薬学
市川 厚・板部洋之・工藤一郎・小林静子
笹津備規・辻坊 裕・山元 弘・榎本武美
- I．生命体の成り立ち 4100円
- II．生命をミクロに理解する（第2版） 5500円
- III．生体防御 3400円
- IV．演習編 市川 厚・板部洋之・榎本武美・笹津備規
高橋 悟・辻坊 裕・山元 弘 4200円

|5| 健康と環境（第2版）6100円
井手速雄・鍛治利幸・永沼 章

|6| 薬 と 疾 病
赤池昭紀・入江徹美・山元俊憲
- IA．薬の効くプロセス（1）薬理（第2版）4200円 栗原順一・比佐博彰
- IB．薬の効くプロセス（2）薬剤（第2版）3200円 山本 昌・渡辺善照
- II．薬物治療（1）（第2版）5600円 小澤孝一郎・徳山尚吾・中村明弘・吉富博則
- III．薬物治療（2）および 薬物治療に役立つ情報（第2版）
5100円 加藤裕久・笹津備規・高野幹久・望月眞弓

|7| 製剤化のサイエンス（第2版）3200円
杉林堅次・須田晃治・平野和行

|8| 医薬品の開発と生産 3400円
須田晃治・戸部 敞・長野哲雄
夏苅英昭・平野和行

|9| 薬学と社会（第3版）3600円
入江徹美・小澤孝一郎・白神 誠
富田基郎・早瀬幸俊

|10| 実務実習事前学習――病院・薬局実習に行く前に 5600円

|11| 病院・薬局実務実習
日本薬剤師会・日本病院薬剤師会
日本医療薬学会と共編
- I．病院・薬局に共通な薬剤師業務 5100円
- II．病院・薬局それぞれに固有な薬剤師業務 4800円

価格は本体価格（消費税別）2013年12月現在